10
11
12
13
15
16
17
18
19
20
21
22
23
24
25
26
27
28

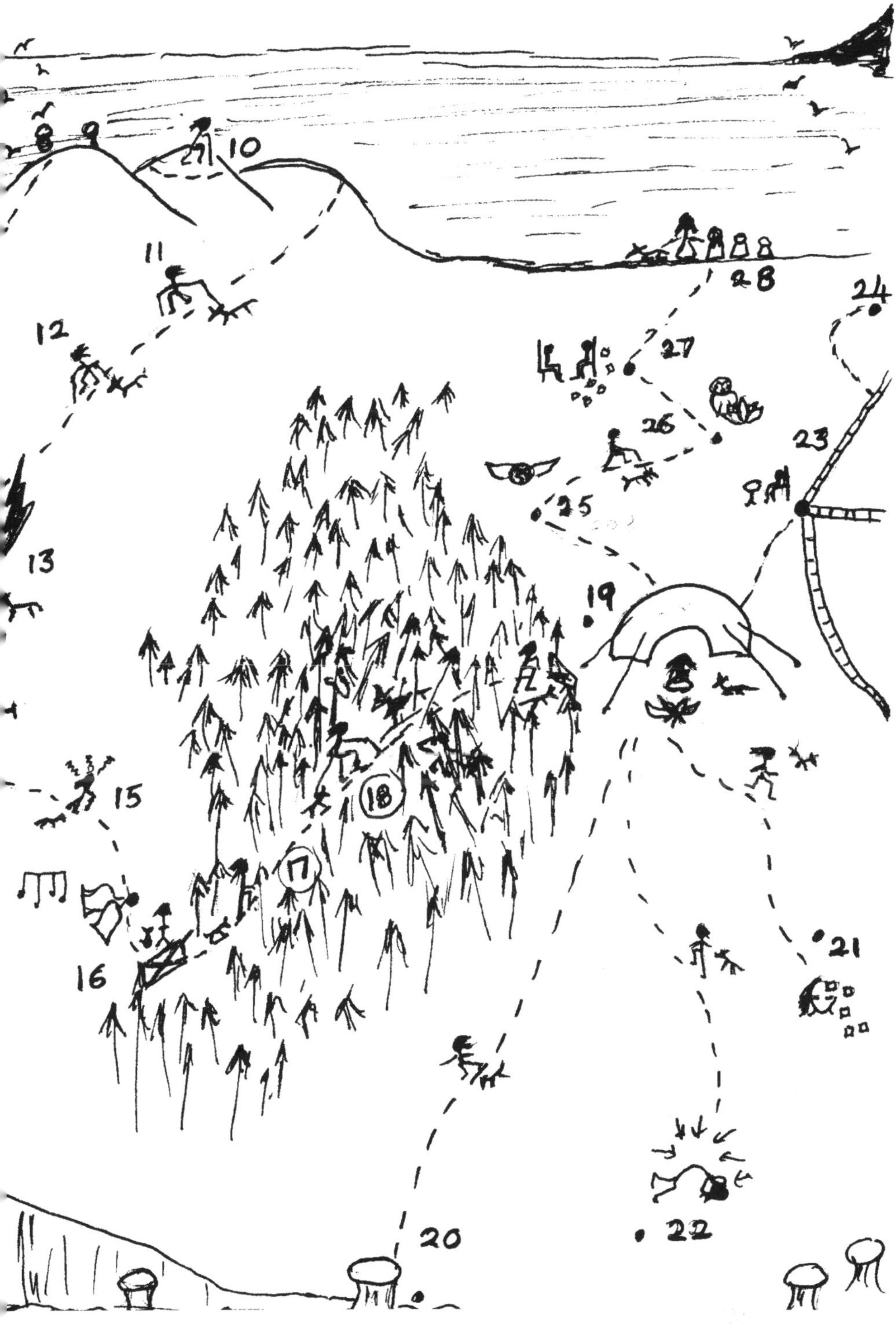

Mindfulness and Stroke
A Personal Story of Managing Brain Injury

© Pavilion Publishing & Media Ltd

The authors have asserted their rights in accordance with the Copyright, Designs and Patents Act (1988) to be identified as the authors of this work.

Published by:
Pavilion Publishing and Media Ltd
Blue Sky Offices
Cecil Pashley Way
Shoreham by Sea
West Sussex
BN43 5FF
Tel: 01273 434 943
Fax: 01273 227 308
Email: info@pavpub.com

Published 2020

All rights reserved. No part of this publication may be reproduced, stored in a retrieval system, or transmitted in any form or by any means, electronic, mechanical, photocopying, recording or otherwise, without prior permission in writing of the publisher and the copyright owners.

A catalogue record for this book is available from the British Library.

ISBN: 978-1-912755-86-8

Pavilion Publishing and Media is a leading publisher of books, training materials and digital content in mental health, social care and allied fields. Pavilion and its imprints offer must-have knowledge and innovative learning solutions underpinned by sound research and professional values.

Editor: Ruth Chalmers, Pavilion Publishing and Media Ltd.
Cover design: Phil Morash, Pavilion Publishing and Media Ltd.
Page layout and typesetting: Phil Morash, Pavilion Publishing and Media Ltd.
Printing: CMP Digital Print Solutions

Contents

About the authors vii
Permissions x
Acknowledgements xi
Foreword xiii
Introduction 1

Part 1: Tsunami in my Brain 5
Chapter 1: The Beginning and the End 7
Chapter 2: Leaving Hospital – Coming Home 15
Chapter 3: There is a Crack in Everything 23
Chapter 4: That's how the Light Gets in 31

Part 2: Cannot Go That Way Again 39
Chapter 5: Over the Rope Bridge 41
Chapter 6: Leave Everything You Know Behind 47
Chapter 7: The Way Lies over the Mountains 55
Chapter 8: Living in the View From My Window 61

Part 3: Over the Mountains 65
Chapter 9: The Cup 67
Chapter 10: Back to Work and Cognitive Testing 71
Chapter 11: Living in my Brain 77
Chapter 12: When Getting Better is Getting Worse 81

Part 4: Down into a New World 85
Chapter 13: Lightning Does Strike Twice 87
Chapter 14: The Landscape Changes 93
Chapter 15: The Edge of the Woods 99
Chapter 16: Leaving Work and the Hum in the Woods 105

Part 5: Into the Woods 111
Chapter 17: Further into the Woods 113
Chapter 18: Wolves in the Woods 117
Chapter 19: Out of the Woods and Building a Camp 121
Chapter 20: Paths that Open and Close 129

Part 6: In the Camp **133**
Chapter 21: Falling Mind...135
Chapter 22: Perception 141
Chapter 23: The Trouble with Travelling 147
Chapter 24: And Change Goes Ever On and On 153

Part 7: Leaving the Camp **161**
Chapter 25: Memory Clinic and Tattoo...............................163
Chapter 26: The Unseen Wounds of Brain Injury 167
Chapter 27: A New Story to be Lived and Breathed 173
Chapter 28: Return to the Beginning..................................179

Chapter 29: Introduction 189
Cognitive Changes After Jody's Stroke..**203**
Chapter 30: Attention 205
Chapter 31: Memory 217
Chapter 32: Planning and Organisation..............................229
Chapter 33: Perception 237
Coming to Terms with a Stroke or Brain Injury **247**
Chapter 34: Loss, Grief and Emotional Distress 249
Chapter 35: The Problem of Reduced Self-Awareness 263
Chapter 36: Identity and Sense of Self 275
Chapter 37: Acceptance..283
Chapter 38: Families..293
Jody's practices 305

About the authors

Jody Mardula is a psychotherapist and supervisor whose professional background in addiction counselling, training and services management culminated in a role as Director of Counselling, Supervision and Training for CAIS, The North Wales Drug and Alcohol Agency, from 1987 to 2006. Jody was also for many years a highly respected practitioner, trainer and examiner in the field of Transactional Analysis (TA).

In 2007 she joined the team at the Centre for Mindfulness Research and Practice at Bangor University, UK, and in 2008 she was appointed the Centre's Director. While serving in this role, Jody suffered her first stroke in 2010 and returned to work after this. She left her post after suffering a second stroke in 2012. She continues to train and teach at a reduced level. She has written numerous journal articles and is the author of chapters on mindfulness in therapy in several edited books.

Dr Frances Vaughan is a clinical neuropsychologist with a background in cognitive and neuropsychology research. After a PhD in cognitive science, and a series of neuropsychology research posts in hospitals and universities around the UK, Frances went on to train as a clinical psychologist in Bangor. She worked in a service for people with dementia, and later, the North Wales Brain Injury Service. At the same time, she had various part-time research and teaching positions at Bangor University. In one of these, she developed and was Director of a clinical neuropsychology training program for clinical psychologists.

More recently, Frances developed a neuropsychological service to support families living with a brain injury, and carried out research into the effects of learning to practice mindfulness after a brain injury. Frances has an Honorary Senior Lectureship at Bangor University.

Mindfulness Audio Recordings

Audio recordings of the mindfulness practices (see p.305) can be downloaded from:

https://www.pavpub.com/mindfulness-and-stroke-resources

Dedication

J.M.

This book is dedicated to helping all those living with the effects of brain injury and stroke, and to those who care for them and are affected by the brain injury of others.

That they may find support and encouragement in bringing mindfulness into their lives, to help them find a way forward.

F.L.V.

To the individuals and families living with stroke and brain injury that I have had the privilege to work with and learn from over the years. I have so often been humbled by your courage, creativity, strength and humour.

And to the vibrant memory of my friend Julie Desborough, who first taught me about the reality of surviving a stroke. More recently, and while dying from cancer, Julie continued to live each day fully, mindfully, and often with her own irrepressible joy.

Permissions

Michael Leunig's poem *When the Heart* used with kind permission.

Quote from T.S. Eliot's *Burnt Norton*, from *Four Quartets* used with permission from Faber & Faber Ltd.

Laurie Lee quote from *As I Walked out one Midsummer Morning* reproduced with permission of Curtis Brown Group Ltd, London on behalf of the Beneficiaries of the Estate of Laurie Lee. Copyright © Laurie Lee 1969.

Extract from *The Little Prince* by Antoine de Saint-Exupéry. English translation copyright © 2000 Richard Howard. First published by Harcourt, Inc 1943. Now published by Egmont UK Limited and used with permission. US rights: Extract from *The Little Prince* by Antoine de Saint-Exupéry. Translated from the French by Richard Howard. Copyright 1942 by Houghton Mifflin Harcourt Publishing Company. Copyright © renewed 1971 by Consuelo de Saint-Exupery, English translation © 2000 by Richard Howard. Reprinted with permission of Houghton Mifflin Harcourt Publishing Company. All rights reserved.

Quotation from 'Anthem' by Leonard Cohen copyright © 1992, Leonard Cohen, used by permission of The Wylie Agency (UK) Limited.

We believe all other poetry extracts to be in the public domain.

Acknowledgements

J.M.

To Samantha Harper – who first taught me about the 'New Normal' that comes with living with a brain injury, and encouraged and supported me in writing a book about it.

To my niece Samantha Babington, for her encouragement that I could do this, and for her book *Serendipity's Secret*.

To my friend and colleague Trish Bartley, who has supported and guided me from start to publication.

To my co-writer Frances Vaughan, for her skill and knowledge in helping me understand my brain injury over the years.

To Heather Melville, who typed and organised the material to get it ready for publication.

To Mark Williams, for his support for my writing this book and for writing the foreword.

To Oliver Turnbull – for his support and encouragement.

To Annee Griffiths and Trish Bartley, for letting me include their poems.

To Chris Pearson, for his support with getting the poetry permissions.

To Neil Rostance, for editing the mindfulness practice recordings.

To all my colleagues at the Centre for Mindfulness, Research and Practice at Bangor University, and to all the participants on the courses that I have taught over the years, and to my supervisees. Thank you all for staying with me through my recovery, and for your continuing faith in me.

So many friends and colleagues down the years, so many people whose lives have touched mine, in whatever way, thank you.

And to all my family – my children and my grandchildren.

F.L.V.

After several years of procrastination and a series of challenging life events, I wrote my neuropsychological commentary far too quickly for comfort. My family and friends were generous enough to rescue and support me through this one last project.

I am particularly grateful to my husband Antony, to the grown-up children I neglected for several months, and to my sister Deb and her wife Liz, who provided a much needed writing retreat.

I am indebted to my neuropsychology colleagues and friends, Dr Rudi Coetzer and Dr Christian Salas, for their patient reading of drafts and support throughout; to Nancy Brown, once my son's English teacher, for her reassurance and invaluable advice on writing style; and to the friends and colleagues who have listened, encouraged and helped in many different ways over the past year. In particular, Rachel Armstrong, Joanna Carson, Dr Sarah Gregory, Dr Gemma Griffiths, Professor Jane Raymond, Dr Estie van Rensberg, Dr Cathryn Roberts, Chrissy Rolfe, Leanne Rowlands, Judith Soulsby and Professor Oliver Turnbull.

Last but not least, my heartfelt thanks to Jody for our extraordinary collaboration, and to the 'team' whose patience and hard work brought this book together; Jody's friends and former colleagues Trish Bartley and Heather Melville, and Darren Reed and Ruth Chalmers of Pavilion Publishing.

Foreword

'I am on a raft... and without words or thought I know that this sea flows into Death and into Life and I may pass down either way. Death feels a peaceful path and Life is noisy, I can hear it, dimly – calling, calling. I know that Death is familiar – that we know how to die...

... And I heard my children calling to me... they wanted me to do something – they wanted me to stay, they wanted me to fight. The raft turned.'

When I read these words for the first time, some years ago now, I knew that this was a book that others needed to read. I have heard people talk of their experiences when, at the very moment of dying, they have returned to life. Jody expresses this in a remarkable way. Her discovery that death is familiar, that we know how to die, is as moving as it is reassuring.

She has had a severe stroke. She describes it with clarity and passion. She tells us about the aftermath: a devastated internal landscape as if a tsunami had ripped through her brain.

'When the waters receded, the landscape of my brain was changed ... I can feel it now as I write – searching... searching for whatever it is that is lost now. And it is exhausting. And my mind is rearranged – I would pick my way then over the cracked mud of the Tsunami buried streets – crawl down the ruined streets of memory. And somehow perhaps find something, maybe a house or room left standing, or hiding somewhere amid the changed landscape. There is a light – familiarity – little organised pockets of memory amid the rubble.'

Then she unfolds the story of a sort of 'recovery' – except that it is not the recovery that she or others might have dreamt of – it is a finding safety in the middle of a strange new world – a coming to know this new world again and again. In the end, her great learning is that there is no such thing as recovery if that means getting back to how things were. Instead, it is about recovering the skill of discovery, curiosity and acceptance of the new self.

'I kept coming back to looking into my eyes – trying to see into and behind the eyes – and saying who are you? Where are you?...'

Her sheer courage in exploring her new, unfamiliar life with relentless inventiveness is astounding. As Trish Bartley says in her beautiful Introduction, what a blessing it is to benefit from Jody's astonishing ability to be mindfully aware of what is unfolding for her as it is happening.

There is so much to learn from this book. First, that virtually all – all – attempts to reassure fall flat. Why do we still try to do it? Bland reassurance is out of our mouths before we can stop it. Why? Is it because we want to say to our dear friend that it doesn't matter that things have changed? That we understand, when clearly we don't? Or that we want desperately to say 'you're still the same'. To us all, she says:

'I am writing about this because managing these basic life tasks can be so terribly hard. And because I found that – for the most part – people simply do not understand that at all … it is difficult for other people perhaps to see the difficulties that are there – they want to see the positives – what is the same. Nothing inside me was the same.'

A second thing we learn is that the effect of a tsunami in the brain goes a long way down into the soul and extends a long way out into the world. Jody shows us how enormously difficult it was to see and get the measure of the awful surprise that the old maps have gone, the roads and pathways have been swept away. This is not the usual form of absentmindedness, forgetting names, or being temporarily overwhelmed by a task that seems a little complex. This is different. More radical. More deeply confusing than anything that most of us have ever experienced.

'The most common response to my sharing these difficulties has always tended to be an assumption that this is just the same as it is for everyone; we all have those 'senior moments' or sudden lapses in memory. But there is something about the quality of this loss with Brain Injury which has a very different quality.'

Next Jody tells us about a form of acceptance which goes much deeper than seeing clearly what is happening. She gives us an example of taking a breathing space when she can't remember something in order to allow it. By 'it', she means the gap created when the road-less emptiness becomes apparent. This is true not only in a shop when the 'it' is an item of food she has meant to buy, but in everyday social life when the information is coming too fast from the friendly chatter of people gathered round table or bed. She says that allowing the gap to be there – not trying to recover the information she knows should have been there – is the only way through.

We learn also of the discovery of jigsaws. Oh! How much even the most caring family and friends can grieve when they see their loved one – someone previously so busy and successful and productive and … (add your own adjective) … doing jigsaws. Here is a lesson for us all – to let go of the 'old normal' here too. For Jody's first-hand account shows us how doing this activity is utterly consoling – she feels it is putting the brain back piece by piece just like the jigsaw. And – while we are about it – let's wonder how we ever fooled ourselves into thinking that we'd ever really, really given up thinking that 'busy, successful, productive' was the aim in life. I can only speak for myself, but I imagine that many of us believe we have got past thinking of productivity as a yardstick for meaning in life, but if you look deeply into yourself when you visit a loved one and you find them playing a 'child's game', see what you notice. Learn from Jody's experience and rejoice with her for jigsaws.

'Frances came to see me and listened – listened to my long, probably rambling accounts of how it was to be me... and she understood what I was saying and explained it to me in neurological and psychological terms that I could understand.'

Frances Vaughan's gentle explanations meant that Jody didn't have to pretend. Neuropsychology was giving the same message as her mindfulness practice: this is how it is now. The joy of this book is that we too get to hear and learn what Jody learned from Frances's deep knowledge of the brain/mind.

Frances writes:
'Imagine being woken up in the middle of the night and finding yourself in a fairground. Surrounded on every side by loud music, bright coloured lights, flashing and chasing around the outside of every ride. Amusement machines making loud noises, some squawking, shrieking, dinging – a huge wall of loud noise. Add to that the sickly-sweet smell of candy floss, a burger grill, hot dogs and frying onions. It sounds like a nightmare – we would all want to hide under the duvet. For Jody, ordinary things such as crossing a busy road or going to a shopping centre were as overwhelming as a fairground... The filter was not working properly, and Jody's senses were flooded and overwhelmed. For her, there was no background noise, only noise ... Because Jody's filter didn't work properly anymore, she often felt overwhelmed and could 'crash' like an overloaded computer.'

In this and other ways, Frances explains clearly how the brain usually works to ensure that we are able to attend to, remember, perceive, organise things around us. She shows how any of these delicate processes can be affected by brain injury and dementia of various kinds. Frances offers us a map of the terrain that we need to understand and begin to navigate the new territory. Because she and Jody trusted each other so well, she is able to speak openly about what was happening to Jody, and to put these experiences into a wider context. She has a special chapter for families, and what they are most likely to need..

Frances realised from the first conversation with Jody how important it is that the 'third person' clinical descriptions of neuropsychology are complemented by the 'first person' lived experience of the person at the heart of the events. The genius of this book is that it offers us both – wisdom from the inside and wisdom from the outside. Jody affirms how helpful it was to be heard by Frances and Frances showed, in her listening, how the best clinicians can come alongside the experience of those they care for.

In keeping faith with their commitment to say honestly what is happening, Jody and Frances share with us the eventual discovery of vascular dementia. And because we are reading her diary, Jody is not only telling us, she is *showing* us. She doesn't hide the gaps and the goings around. As she says, she used to be able to hold in mind the book and the structure of its separate parts and chapters…..but '…*now, I cannot hold them all in memory at one time. I am quite likely to wake up tomorrow not knowing I have written any of this. Unless I have left myself some notes, I could well start all over again.*'

And with stark clarity '…*I am going to stop now, I am tired, and I feel too tired to write a lot of notes. I will just put one note on top of the PC and one by the kettle in the kitchen saying "you are typing a Chapter near the end".*'

This is not a romantic story of wonderful resilience constantly winning the battle against desperation. Jody is utterly honest: '*I wanted to be back as I had been. They wanted me to be back as I had been*'. The work, as she defines it for herself, is to see and 'hold close' these longings within the larger reality of what was actually happening.

Jody's story in this book began with being close to death. But the raft turned, and she returned to life – but, in so many ways, not the same one. It is an extraordinary witness to Jody's own persistence, to Frances' wise encouragement, and to the gentle help of her family and many friends (re-read the Acknowledgements and give thanks), that this book is here for us. It is a remarkable gift for us all, so that we, when this happens to us or to our loved ones, may discern the courage to discover new ways of living life.

Mark Williams
Emeritus Professor of Clinical Psychology, University of Oxford

Introduction

You hold in your hands an unusual book. In many ways, it is an intimate invitation into the mind and the heart of someone who has experienced what she calls a 'tsunami' in her brain, a life-threatening and devastating stroke, leaving her with a significant brain injury. This was followed sometime later by another bleed into her brain, and later still, a diagnosis of vascular dementia.

Jody Mardula has written this book a little like a personal journal. Indeed much of her writing has been transferred directly from reflections within her many notebooks – as have her lovely illustrations, which have been drawn anew for this book, or adapted from the many drawings she does on an everyday basis.

As you read this, you may sometimes find that the tenses can seem a bit muddled, or the time sequences have changed. Most of it reads as if in the present – happening now – and yet it often refers to things just gone. Jody vividly describes and directly involves us in all the different ways she has experienced life over the nine years after her first catastrophic stroke – which, with all that followed, left her with a life-changing brain injury.

So she writes almost in the form of stream of consciousness – a little like those exercises where you are invited to keep writing with your pen on the paper. I believe you will find, as you read her words, that you will become more and more familiar with how it must be to be inside her mind.

This is both extraordinary and insightful. For those of you who have perhaps experienced something similar, her descriptions may be familiar. If that is the case, then Jody will be speaking directly to you, which is one of the heartfelt wishes that she has for this book. I know that she hopes that her words will offer comfort to people who have been through something similar to her.

For those of us who haven't experienced anything close to this, it may describe a brand new world. This does not always make comfortable reading. In places, Jody does not mince her words. She expresses frustration a number of times when people suggest 'helpful' solutions to her; or when she is offered soothing platitudes such as 'we all do that too'; or when told that in time she will recover. As time has passed, we have slowly come to realise that this simply does not help – and that the best and kindest way is simply to listen to what she is telling us and be there with her in that.

Jody has written this book over many years. Things have gradually changed for her over that time. When her first stroke happened, she needed to be in hospital for a period of time and her adjustment to life at home was considerable on her return. Eventually, she was well enough to return to work – to a senior university post, heading up a leading mindfulness centre in the UK.

Indeed, her background is impressive. She was a senior psychotherapist, trainer and supervisor. She was someone well known, highly skilled and very well respected in her field, who wrote articles and contributed to books – and who had a certain originality about the way she worked and trained others to work. People loved learning from her, not least for the sometimes mischievous and slightly irreverent way that she had. We enjoyed and continue to enjoy her somewhat eccentric ways. She is undoubtedly much loved – not just by her family and friends, but also by those she trained, taught and worked with.

In due course, Jody became involved in mindfulness-based approaches and took over the directorship of the Centre for Mindfulness, Research and Practice (CMRP) at Bangor University, at a time when significant research was happening. Her role and what she contributed at this time was also significant. She brought with her some strong leadership and management skills – and managed to form and consolidate a staff team, which could run the centre in a way that was much needed.

So there was an extended period of time when many of the key roles in the CMRP were filled by people appointed by Jody, who brought her keen sense of what was needed to deciding who should fill the post. Then her first tsunami stroke happened, and things were never quite the same again. She did her best, as she describes, to keep the show on the road, and in some ways she succeeded, but it was hard for her. It was also hard for others at work to adjust to this new Jody, whom everyone hoped would recover and return to how she had been. She describes this so well. But sadly that never quite happened.

She wrote this book with a strong desire to benefit others. She hopes that it will offer tangible support to people who have experienced brain injuries like hers. She has greatly relied on a long established mindfulness practice to help her manage this time – and she has been very resourceful and creative in the way that she has developed her practice to form short, simple exercises that align with what she needed. She has shared these with you in this book. I know she is excited to discover whether they will be of use to other stroke and brain injury affected people. She hopes very much that they will.

Her stories and use of metaphor are typical of Jody's quick creativity. The map that she created helps us to understand the journey she has been on, which she describes in her writing. The map and her journey metaphors have also helped her make meaning of some painful and some joyous times – and much else in between.

Understandably, there have been people behind her who have helped her bring this book into being. It is important for you to understand, as a reader of this book, that she has increasingly needed others to help her remember. A small team has supported her – typing up her writing, scanning her pictures, and so on. None of this would have happened without Jody's vision and incredible commitment to writing this book.

In the second half of this book, Frances Vaughan writes about the neuropsychological implications of stroke and brain injury. Her writing offers special value and insight into our understanding and knowledge. The explanations and suggestions in her chapters and in the 'Neuro Notes' at the end of each of Jody's sections are quite unique. Frances has vast knowledge in this field. She is an academic researcher of long standing, with many learned articles behind her, and is therefore well placed to write in this way. We, her readers, can be assured that she absolutely knows what she is telling us.

One of Jody's challenges, especially in the early days, was her difficulty in finding books that spoke to her of her experience. This is the book that she wanted to find, I imagine – rich in professional knowledge and wisdom and also in direct personal experience. Jody and Frances have long held the vision of producing a two-part book like this – jointly written by the one affected and by the one offering professional expertise and care. This book offers us a unique and unusual glimpse into this important area of stroke and brain injury (and also vascular dementia), which affects so many thousands of people every year. I strongly commend this book to you.

Trish Bartley

Part 1: Tsunami in my Brain

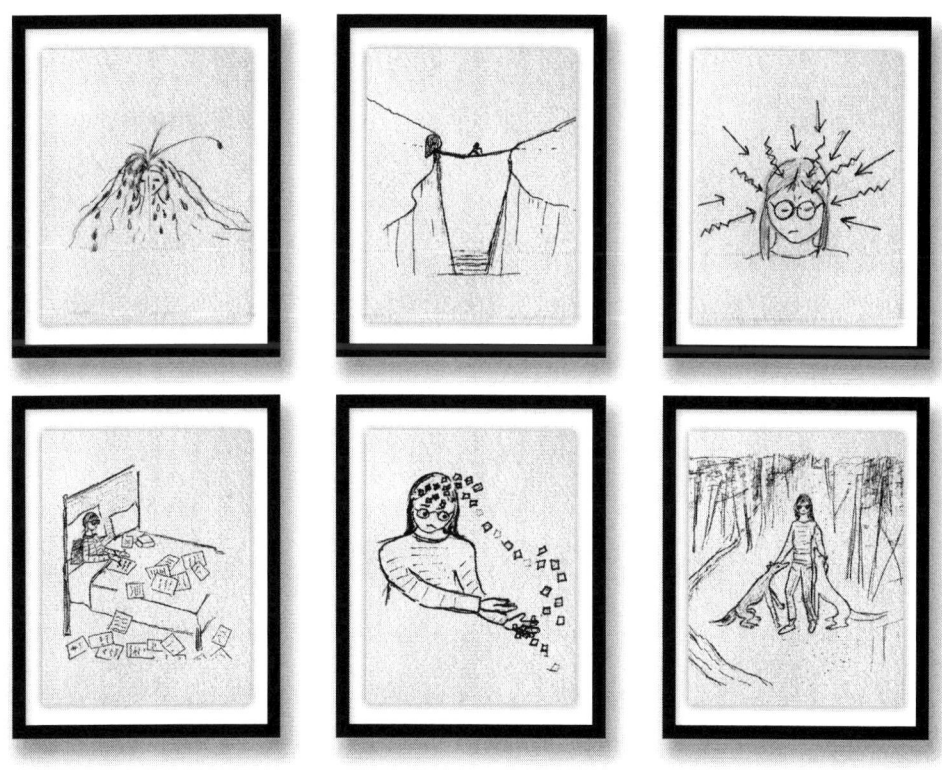

Chapter 1: The Beginning and the End

A volcano lay dormant in the mind – emptying a waterfall of blood – sweeping away – erasing the topsoil – like flood waters – leaving the land – the solid rock – when the water recedes – the landscape of the mind is drained.

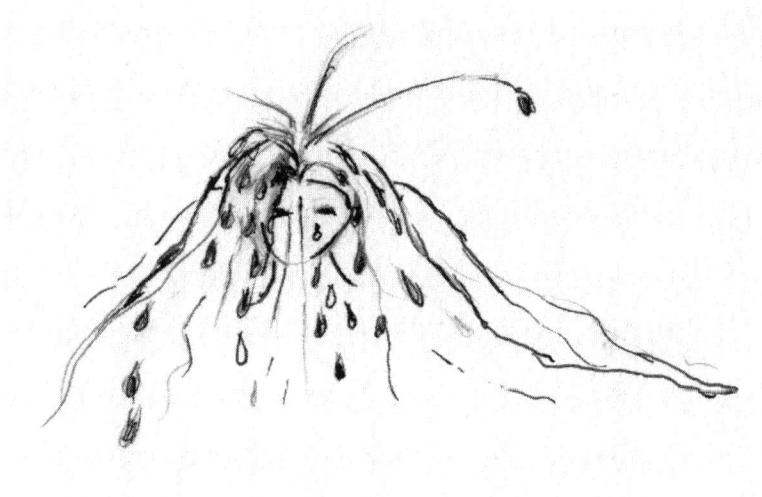

I am packing to fly to an island that I spent time on with my first husband… it seemed a long time ago – 1967. We were in our early twenties and travelling around Spain in a battered old Morris van. It was blue. I was pregnant with my first child.

I had long planned to return to this island. It was one of those places and times that stand out in the memory as significant in our lives.

Now, 43 years later, I am living in North Wales. I am Director of the Centre for Mindfulness Research and Practice at Bangor University. I am a Mindfulness Teacher and a Psychotherapist. I have three grown up children.

Chapter 1: The Beginning and the End

On Thursday 5 August 2010 I was enjoying myself packing for my trip – making lists – sorting out what had to be done before I went – and making a small pile of what to take with me, when I noticed I had quite a strong, sudden headache. I often have a bit of a headache in the morning so did not think much of it, and I continued to gather things for my journey.

Then, as I come out of the bathroom I suddenly cannot see properly – I feel a rush of very intense nausea – I stumble and a searing, stabbing pain shoots through my head and then settles into a solid throbbing pain… the nausea increases… I vomit – projectile vomiting – a strange far away thought amid the pain, that I know these symptoms… our daughter had just these symptoms 42 years ago when she had meningitis and then hydrocephalus as a baby – the pressure on her brain causing these conditions… and I thought, there is something wrong… but I was trying to get back to the bedroom – I had to finish packing – I had to get to our island. I could feel cold water running, running in my head. There is such pain in my head.

The pain got worse, I couldn't see and then it was as if I heard a voice – insistent – 'this is your brain – this is urgent you have to DO something – phone someone… phone'… and I know I passed out… when I came to I was lying at the top of the stairs outside the bathroom… and right beside me was the phone. Blackness is closing in…

There are a series of coincidences here – my daughter's father had died of a brain haemorrhage – a subarachnoid aneurysm. It seemed to be his voice telling me something was wrong. Because of my daughter's brain damage from childhood she had difficulties in seeing small numbers and making phone calls so we always kept the telephone at the top of the stairs by her bedroom door – it had very large buttons to press so that she could easily call people – or ask for help – and even though she left home more than 10 years ago that phone was still there. Otherwise, I don't think I could have called for help – and there was this insistent voice in my head – call – call, and so I picked the receiver up – and because I could not see anything, I felt my way to what I thought was the 9 and pressed 9 9 9.

I could feel the water flowing more strongly in my head and down the back of my neck – it was cold – I felt so sick and my head hurt so much, but it was very distant – I could only see shapes. I didn't feel frightened – I did not feel alone – I felt a sense of worry about my family – I knew I needed to stay awake until help got to me. I must stay here. I must stay here.

I remember a voice down the phone, and telling her my address – I knew she was trying to keep me talking – strangely I knew what she was doing and why – but I couldn't do it – more words wouldn't come – it was too much energy – there was a stiffening around my jaw… a deep lassitude… falling… sinking… sinking.

I felt an extraordinary calm. A confidence that whatever happened, there was no right or wrong – no good or bad – there was no fear. I had a sense of trust and acceptance, I think. It was as though I was observing myself from a distance – why was there a waterfall at the back of my head? I could hear it.

I must have dropped in and out of consciousness because then I heard some sort of crash downstairs and the ambulance men were there – calling to me – 'she's up here' – carrying me – talking to me – looking at me – kind voices – insistent voices. Hands lifting me. I could see myself being lifted and wheeled out into the street.

I think I knew I was in an ambulance – in and out of knowing – drifting – moving – darkness – someone was holding my hand – I could feel the contact.

And it was as if I sank deeper – a gentle falling away – falling away to a place – mostly – of not knowing. Now and then the insistence of someone – now and then the intrusion of awareness of the pain that I knew was always there – sudden noise – pain of movement then darkness – a warm and, I think, gentle darkness – as I recall. And I wanted them to just let me go… And who knows how much or how little we recall of anything in these places…

I think I had drifted a long way away then – sometimes in and sometimes out of my body. Voices came from far away – sometimes I was aware of being moved – rocked on trolleys – sailing along corridors – dimly aware of walls – moving – lights – aware of the contact of my body on the trolley. At one end of the corridor I was in, there was a light that was receding – I knew it was home – my life – my world – receding farther… I was being pushed further and further away from it… at the other end another light… softer – restful – inviting – and I knew that if I let myself just let go and sink into sleep the pain would go – so tempting – to rest there… further and further away. And I knew that somehow the other light was my life – if I wanted to go back there I would have to fight, to choose – a choice between pain and peace. I so wanted to go towards the peace – to let go…

And I was drifting between the two lights – far out to sea, leaning towards the resting…

And I float on a wide, wide, deep sea beneath a huge, huge sky – nothing but still movement – I am on a raft… and without words or thought I know that this sea flows into Death and into Life and I may pass down either way. Death feels a peaceful path and Life is noisy, I can hear it, dimly – calling, calling. I know that Death is familiar – that we know how to die.

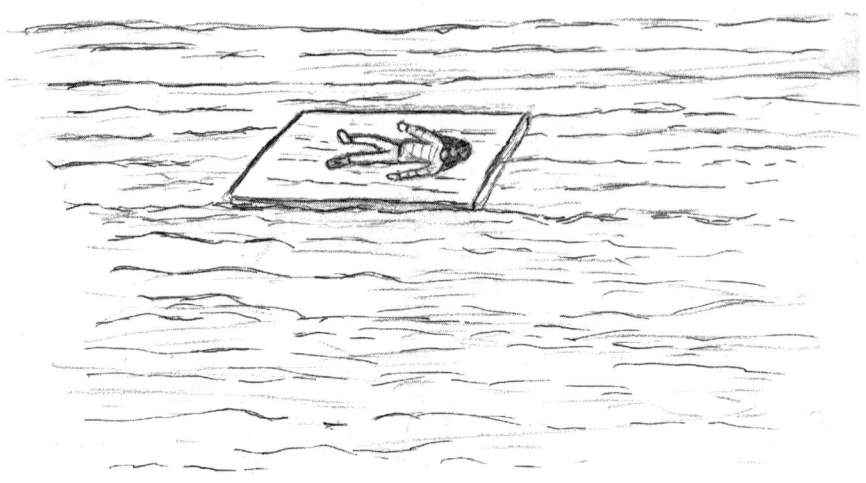

And I heard my children calling to me – my son F and youngest daughter D – my son's voice loud – insistent – 'Mum, Mum' – and I felt his hand – felt my daughter's hand – 'Mum, Mum' – calling to me. And I began to fight – somehow I knew it wasn't time to go yet – they were insistent – they wanted me to do something – they wanted me to stay, they wanted me to fight. The raft turned.

I felt the touch, of others' hands
The feel of others – near
A reassuring connection
To a world no longer here

I know now how important those voices and hands were and are. The feel of the presence of others – the contact of the touch of a hand – soothing – comforting – urging – a sense of not being alone, of contact.

I don't really remember much of anything until, I suppose, some hours – or days – later. A vague sense of people standing around me – huge machines – bending over me. I was in a Hospital Ward now looking up – and they were there, either side of me – hands – and nurses and tubes and a terrible, terrible pain in my head and it seemed everywhere and all I could think, I remember, was 'why have I been run over by a steamroller?' Everything hurt. I couldn't do anything. I didn't know what had happened.

And they were always there through that first waking, my children – my son F and youngest daughter D – even when they had gone I could feel the imprint of their hands on mine, pulling me back – and then other hands – family – my daughter-in-law K and son-in-law C, then dear friends – and my eldest daughter H – although she could not come and see me, she was there too.

And I knew for the first time from the inside what she had been through – as a baby – through her life – she was there too.

And sometimes when it was quiet – when everyone had gone – I felt the presence and voices of other loved ones who had gone. And always I think I was with myself.

But I was held – supported by whatever I was lying on – by voices and hands and the presence of others. By my sense of what was supporting – holding me. By my breath. I knew my breath was there. I was in a familiar yet strange place, hovering between the known and the unknown. But even then – and, I realised later, through the procedures and operation I had been through – that awareness of being supported and grounded had been there, as well as a dim awareness that I was always accompanied by my breath. The sense of having been on a raft persisting – supported – breathing.

And – much later – I realised that this had been my Mindfulness Meditation Practice, which I had sat and practised most days for many years. Where the first mindfulness practices I had learned were to feel the contact of my body with whatever was supporting it – floor – chair – meditation cushion. And how to simply feel and watch the movement of the breath as it moves in and out of the body. To come into the present moment. And to stay with that moment – to let whatever is here to be here – not to fight it.

And gradually I could move more, eat a little and learn to tolerate the pain and when to take medication, when to eat… And I knew, somewhere without thoughts, that something had changed.

I was wired up to things – as I became more aware I noticed how uncomfortable that was – began to get restless when my family were not there – I missed the feel of their hands… And I began to imagine their hands were there, to notice how my hands felt – and it was as if I could feel the imprint of their hands and all those hands – family, friends, ambulance men, nurses, doctors that had brought connection and comfort even when I was barely conscious. And I began to use my mindfulness.

HANDS PRACTICE
I felt the sense of my hands resting on the sheets.
I could feel the softness of the sheets beneath the hands.
Breathing into the hands.
And deliberately imagined the sense of hands.
The remembered sense of their hands resting on mine.
Lying there, on my raft bed, breathing into my hands.
Connected, I was not alone.

And later, when they had taken all the tubes out of my right hand – *I moved one hand to rest on the other and brought kindness and connection into my practice.*

Then they began to get me out of bed – and it was then that the changes, that something huge had happened to me, became apparent. Not being able to walk unaided – before I left hospital having a Walking Stick… The strangeness of going to a bathroom – not remembering how to turn a tap on – the strangeness of the feel of the water – realising I knew what to do – how to wash – but it was all so complicated. Brushing my teeth – how would I ever do this unaided… and then I remember so clearly the first moment that I looked into the mirror.

Even now I cannot remember that without a huge surge of emotion – bewilderment – shock – who was that… I knew it must be 'me' but it wasn't – it didn't look anything like me – though as I looked closer I remember thinking 'ah yes, this is like me… but not'. And then looking curiously closer and deep into my eyes – and I knew this was 'me' but I was not the same. I kept coming back to looking into my eyes – trying to see into and behind the eyes – and saying who are you? Where are you?

(And I still do this now – writing almost exactly six years from the date of the bleed. Only now I am getting to know the territory of 'me' – I am six (not 70) years old – and I have a six-year-old's 'new eyes that can look with wonder at the world'.)

Strangely, it seemed I knew who I was – mother, daughter, sister, friend… but also I knew that I had been changed. It was frightening and I was also a little curious… Where was I? Who was I? How are things going to be now?

I didn't know it then but this changed sense of self was going to be one of the major features of my life and recovery… somehow it changed everything.

So I was up and walking around with my stick a little – still often in so much pain – so exhausted – every step such an effort of attention and movement – my head hurt – my whole body felt battered, the lights of the ward still seemed over bright – the walls moved strangely but I was acclimatising… beginning to open to this new world.

And I learnt that I had had a Sub Arachnoid Haemorrhage – that an Aneurysm had burst in my head – sending blood surging around the brain – and they had inserted a coiling through the artery into the site of the bleeding to encourage the blood to clot – and the bleeding to stop.

There would be some consequences, though no one really knew what they would be. I had been 'lucky' – I could have died.

There were to be many consequences. But mostly they have not been the ones I, or it seemed anyone much, might have imagined. It is what may seem like the 'little' things of life – the changes in personality and sense of self – the subtle differences in ability – the unpredictability of memory – the learning – because nobody can tell you about it – of the 'New Normal' – a wonderful phrase that I learnt from a dear friend who I met some four years after my Haemorrhage and who had herself lived for 18 years with the effects of what I came to know as an Acquired Brain Injury. We shared a knowing that other people do not know – they look for you to be 'the same' – a knowing of a New Normal. We had a New Normal. I loved that.

I know that I have been incredibly fortunate in the support I have had, the friends and colleagues I have, the wonderful family I have. That I worked with people who knew about Mindfulness – who knew about the psychological effects of Brain Injury. The people who have worked with me as I returned to work – to teaching mindfulness – Frances, who has contributed to this book and helped me to make sense of the changes I have experienced – to begin to see how we can use them to hopefully be of help to others.

And it has perhaps been my Mindfulness Practice that has supported me in even the hardest – loneliest – most painful moments – and it has been my mindfulness practice too that has enabled me to really live all of this experience – and understand it – and that is why I am writing this book. Because although I was extremely lucky that I had this practice to turn to during my haemorrhage and afterwards – Mindfulness could be such a helpful tool for carers – for family – and to teach to others with Brain Injury.

A BRIEF MINDFULNESS BREATHING PRACTICE
Bring your attention to noticing that you are lying here on the bed.
Notice the contact of the body with the bed.
Feel the contact of the body with the bed.
And feel the breath as it moves in and out of your body.
Noticing as you breathe in.
And noticing as you breathe out.
Breathing In. Breathing Out.
Breathing In. Breathing Out.
And now bringing that breathing practice to a close.
And now coming out of that practice and carrying on with what you are doing.

Chapter 2: Leaving Hospital – Coming Home

How might I draw a slipping mind. It is as though a slide of mud builds up and then slips – taking my thoughts and memories with it until they lie, jumbled at the bottom – still there – but coated in the silt.

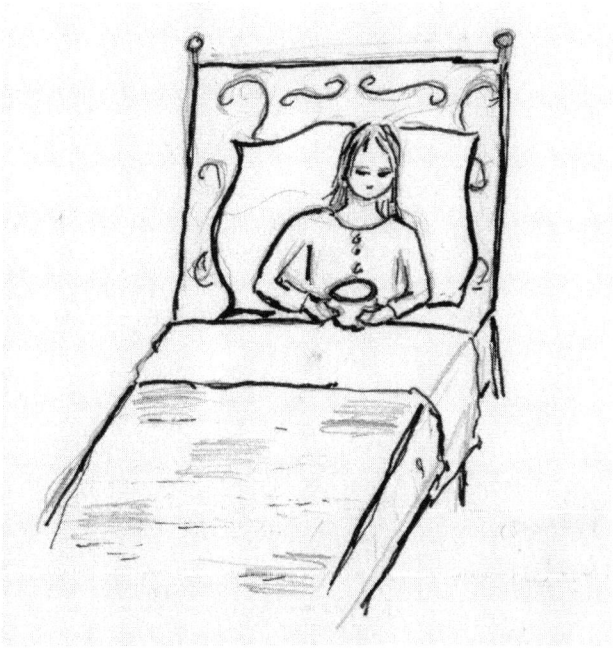

My family came to get me to take me home. I felt bewildered, a mix of excitement and wanting to be home and just not sure what it all would be like. I was to go in the car with my son, F, driving. I know he drove so carefully, not particularly fast, but for me just being outside getting into the car felt strange, TERRIFYING, huge, it was dark and cold.

The journey was another taste of what I could expect for a while – it felt as though we were hurtling along... the street lights and motorway lights were unbearably bright and seemed to be moving towards me like arrows... the sides of the roads falling forwards towards us in the hurtling car. Everything seemed huge. I knew I was safe with F and yet was so terrified... after a while I shut my eyes and just dealt with the strange sensation of movement – the loud noise of the moving car. I didn't recognise anything though when we got to the tunnels – (where I live has tunnels on the roads through the mountains at each end of the village) – I began to realise this is home.

Then we went into the tunnel and I was completely overwhelmed again, by the walls falling in and the glaring, moving, stabbing lights surrounding me and the road with the tunnel side rising up around it seemed to rise up as if about to hit us or I expected us to be thrown over backwards. This theme of difficulty in how I perceived what was around me in movement has persisted, though nothing was ever as overwhelming as that first journey.

I arrived Home – at my House – I felt a bit battered, but I remember how relieved I was – this was home – even if when I went through the front door into my house and stood in the hall – it all looked different. It looked like the wrong house but felt like the right one.

Later that night, when they had got me into my lovely comfy bed in my thankfully familiar bedroom, I felt so loved and cared for. There were flowers and cards everywhere – my family would stay for a while to help me settle into whatever life was now – there were so many messages from friends. I realised how lucky I was – and that if I was going to manage whatever the changes were to be I needed to just be grateful and to simply be in each moment, deal with whatever was here right now and not let myself start wishing things were different or alarming myself with thoughts of what might go wrong.

Mostly that attitude has seen me through… though there have been plenty of times when I have done anything but!

But as I went through the next few weeks, gradually getting up, finding out how to get down stairs, where things were, how to wash, so much I had taken for granted, the full realisation of the changes began to dawn. My children would have to return to normal life, F and K were only down the road, D and C would have to return to life in Brighton soon… I needed to learn to manage alone. Lots of people came… social workers, occupational therapists, to put up things to make it easy for me to get around and do things… sort the house out – check how I was for a while.

I would have to manage my own medication, pain relief, making food, shopping. It all felt bewildering. But mostly I immediately forgot about all this – and that of course also became a huge problem – there is so much we have to remember just to stay alive and manage day by day.

And then everything settled down and I was alone – lots of visits – but I think I welcomed the times of aloneness… I had to find a way to get on with my life as I was now… I had to find out who I was now… and then that ever present question – I had to find out WHO I was now.

I think if I had realised how changed I was I would have been terrified – but I didn't – I wasn't really looking forward. There was only NOW.

In those early days at home, I felt stunned, as if some great power had picked me up and shaken me until everything in my head – my memories – how I saw – heard – and felt – how things looked, were shaken loose and left in a jumbled heap.

Some things I think were gone – lost forever as they were swept away on the tidal wave of blood. Others were hidden – buried.

For a long time my senses seemed all muddled up. And if I am tired enough that still happens today.

The image of a great biblical type flood came to me. It was as though a river had washed through my mind – swelling and falling in torrents around my brain – breaking its banks, widening – eroding and drowning the surrounding land. Before I had taken for granted that ability to, without thinking about it, turn my attention to searching my memory – or thinking about something and making links with existing knowledge, past experience, imagining how something might unfold in the future, based on previous life knowledge. As automatic as putting one step in front of another and walking.

Now I didn't know where to turn. That sense of the brain as a muscle, a solid object was in a way I had not thought of before – and finding it was not responding – like an arm suddenly frozen, unable to be moved – or even felt. Or I would pick up some thoughts or memories but so often they were disconnected – as I grasped something I might feel it slip away from me – leaving a gap.

Simple everyday tasks seemed to come back quite easily – cleaning my teeth – washing my hands and face. But even these were changed experiences – I was completely focussed on the task and whole experience – and if one element was missing, for example, the soap was not where I expected it to be, then everything went blank. I tried and tried to think where soap might be (or the toothpaste or towel or whatever). Exhausting, distressing.

I learned to notice – stop – and leave that task, go and rest, and it would probably come back. People say, 'oh I do that all the time' or 'we all do that'. But the quality is completely different. There are different qualities to 'everyday memory slips' when tired or with too much going on – or 'menopausal lapses' or 'senior moments'. Brain Injury slips and blanks come from a different place – for me they came from the absence of information or a known pathway. There was no known pathway.

Chapter 2: Leaving Hospital – Coming Home

The image of a Tsunami of the Brain came to me – about five months later after I came home – listening to the radio – hearing the reporting of a description of the terrible Japanese earthquake and tsunami that had swept over the land washing away whole cities. And as I listened, it was as if I saw blood red waters rising up and sweeping through my brain – swirling waters of blood – ripping up memories and knowledge and how the world looked – hurling it all about – and how when the waters receded, the landscape of my brain was changed.

That is what I could feel in my head, nothing but the screaming of the blood rushing through the territory of my brain, rearranging things, sweeping away familiarity – objects destroyed – moved – changed.

Later finding familiar objects and landmarks had been moved, lying half buried in different unmarked streets. Sinking into thick walls of red mud – clogging streets and buildings that remained.

And when the waters subsided the landscape of my mind had been changed. How things looked – tasted – felt – sounded. And slowing everything down so that everything around me seemed loud, people talked so quickly, often I just heard a jumble of words, I could not keep up. Sometimes it was as if people were shouting a jumble of mixed up words at me in another language.

So when I first came home – first tried to walk, turned as we do to my brain, my thoughts, my memory, for guidance, for answers – there was little there – most of it had been eradicated, buried, moved or changed. I felt alone. So alone, because I – I was not there. I was not with me. I 'knew' that, I couldn't explain it – indeed, it has been some years in the understanding.

So I retreated for long periods of time to the one place that seemed safe – quiet – my bed, my bedroom. I have a huge Victorian bed – quite high – nothing could have been better (although I had to stand on a stool to get on it). And I looked out over my wonderful bedroom view – across the sea – sky. Just watching the view – clouds moving – sea – birds – weather. Supported. Breathing. A place where I could pause and come back to home. And gradually rebuild – starting with the simple tasks – the landscape of my mind.

Bit by bit a pattern emerged. My daughter went back to Brighton – for a long time she called every day – and my son and daughter-in-law were close by – there was support and visits. Everyone seemed keen to get me up – out – doing things. I remember people saying things like 'you'll soon be back to normal'. I remember even back then not taking much notice of all this, I knew that things could not be as they were before and, although there has been much I wish sometimes I could still do, I never really wanted to be the same as before. I had changed, I knew that, and in a way I was curious – I wanted to get on with finding out how to be with me now and explore this new world.

I learned how to do most everyday tasks, but very slowly – very repetitively. Everything had to be in its place. The tea canister – the cups – the milk – the biscuits. I labelled where things were – if for any reason anything wasn't there, or had been moved, that could feel like a disaster – I didn't seem to have the ability to search – to look into or under things.

It reminded me of my children – that wonderful stage when they are very young and first realise a toy is under the blanket – or this round red wooden block goes into that round hole. But I am going ahead of myself here! This is advanced stuff! If it was in front of me it was there. If it wasn't then it didn't exist.

All these things, although I came to understand them and to adapt to work with them, have mostly stayed with me. And it has led me to change the way I live, organise my house, my activities. Unless I can establish an easy and obvious place to put something and then automatically go to it when I want it again, things are lost forever – or could be. Once an article of clothing, for instance, is in the wardrobe or in a drawer, it may never come out again. So – this stage was about learning – going back to the beginning.

An important learning was getting out. A new stick was brought for me – I learned how to get up and down stairs sitting down – and I went out with two helpers to learn to walk outside! There is a handy rail down my garden path that was there for my daughter H when she was at home – so that was helpful.

And then we were in the street – and it looked so strange – it took me a long time to get used to how strange everything looked – the same but different – and the tendency of walls and trees and lampposts to move. I had two sticks to start with and then one – it was hard to coordinate them and I was shocked at how difficult and different it was to walk – my right leg seemed to do something odd. I remember coming back inside and they made me tea and I was so utterly exhausted. And gradually I learned to walk just a little way up and down the road – with my helpers and then – exciting and scary – alone.

There were so many things – every activity had to be approached in a new way – I could not remember where anything was or how to turn anything on. I had to learn it all – as well as walking and all the things we do without thinking. Washing and dressing are some of the most complicated things imaginable (it took me five years before I could wash my hair without flooding the bathroom and soaking myself from head to foot!)

Chapter 2: Leaving Hospital – Coming Home

Some weeks later I wrote in my Journal *'4.30am and between pills and I am alone now, and meant to be "getting better" whatever that means! My family, drawn for a while from their lives into mine, have gone now. I need to let them go back into their lives and I need to go into mine – to find out what that is now, what I am now. Who I am now. I need to open to my friends, I know I need support. Somehow I need to find out how to survive now.*

All my resources seem stripped away, I cannot drive or even walk beyond the street at the moment. How will I shop, buy food, get to the Doctors etc? I need to find new ways but I feel at a very low ebb this morning.

In a way this is a bit like being new born in a different body. Harder to be in. I cannot trust it to endure.

When I try to bring attention to something – remember something – I experience a sensation of slabs of my brain slipping, shifting in my head. I seem to feel it moving in the same way I might be aware that I am moving an arm – and I have never experienced this sense of the brain being a part of my body before – not in this way. It is slightly scary.'

Mostly I rested – to just lie still was so restful – to just watch the weather, the changing light as day turned to night, the stars coming out. I had no awareness of time – time passing – there was only this moment. And there is a great comfort in that. I think now this perhaps is a protecting factor in brain injury, and in any deep trauma – we need to be able to just lie fallow – like the wounded animal we are at these times.

As the flood waters subsided, the landscape of my mind was changed. How things looked, felt, sounded. Everything was slowed down around me – other people seem to move in a faster, louder world – seemed to speak so quickly – I couldn't follow them. What I often heard was a shouted jumble of words.

There was a gradual knowing that however much support I had, I was alone – and slowly, after a few weeks, I began to want to go further afield.

My first excursion was in the evening – I remember the familiarity of the quality of the light, the birds calling as they came in to roost – jackdaws settling into their night trees around me. And I went slowly up the field at the back – leaning heavily on my stick. So aware – aware of just this moment now – all the tiny movements that I had to make just to move a leg – the smell of grass and earth – birds – warm, caressing air.

I didn't go far – probably a five-minute walk – I remember it was dark when I got home. And that was one of those moments of fear – I could not find how to switch lights on. I just went back to my bed – my safe place – and watched and listened to the night sky. To just breathe with the pain – pain increased, I noticed, with activity. It was no different to any other sensation that came and passed by – it was just that it was an unpleasant experience.

I think I began to see that I just had to follow this new road – there were no options of going back or sideways – only forwards. I knew I would go further now.

I have to use this as a gateway. The gate is open now. Often disguised and hidden but it is there. It is covered with thorns and brambles but I have to cut through. Feel the cuts and tears and keep going. I need to trust though I am afraid – I feel too weak. Do I have the courage to walk through? I don't know the way.

I think I can only go through alone though, find some inner strength.

And this was the point where I was beginning to find my way through all these bewildering changes. I knew that I no longer fit in my life as it had been. The inner world of my moment-by-moment experience – hours just watching the sea changing, the clouds moving across the sky, the birds circling, landing on the roofs and the telegraph wires – the colours of the leaves, the sound of them moving in a breeze – these were more real to me now than the things that used to occupy my days and my mind.

And I think I knew that it was through that inner world that my change, my way to being in the bewildering world outside, would be found.

Chapter 3: There is a Crack in Everything

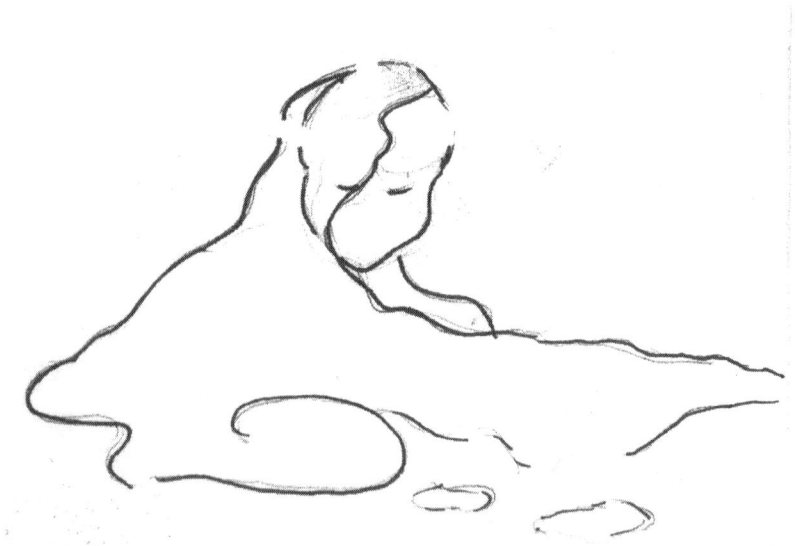

Gradually, as I rested, I became accustomed to the slow pace – learned to keep coming back to the sense of safety in my body – feeling the weight of my body on my bed, through the feet on the floor and increasingly, now, propped up by a huge pile of lovely blue and orange cushions on my sofa in the front room.

I began to come downstairs for a few hours each day. A different view of the sea and garden – the pictures and books and in the corner, the television – which visitors were often keen to turn on for me as something to 'do'. In the end I covered it – I could not bear how quickly the images moved and the bright light of the screen. The words were mixed and did not make sense. There was enough going on in my head just getting used to sitting quietly in a room without more going on.

It felt exciting to be 'downstairs' and I was learning what I could do and not do, what I wanted to do – and I seemed to suddenly want to play a card game of Patience – strangely I could remember very clearly my Mother teaching me this particular game when I was quite young. She used to sit and play it a lot. My son found me the cards and I could remember – as I spread them out – just this one game – where you of course play it over and over, sometimes getting the outcome that all the cards are used (winning) and sometimes some being left (losing).

It was so exciting – and now I realise that what I was able to do was to simply put my attention on the movement of each card and enjoy the process – no urge to get anywhere – no more pleasure in 'winning' than 'losing' – just playing. I was obsessed with this – it was like being hungry – I felt that my brain needed this in the same way my body needed food.

So my day changes – I played patience sometimes in bed and usually now on the sofa. And I sometimes listened to the radio – not music – words, I didn't really need to understand them – or know what the programme was – just listening to words.

And of course all this WAS helping my brain, I could FEEL it. I was re-acclimatising myself to words and sound, to numbers – and repetitive tasks became important – I could do them and I enjoyed it. This was very much at variance with how I had been – I would normally quite quickly have tired of this.

And I began to be curious about going a bit further than the end of the street for my walks and so we set out (my stick and I) to walk down the hill, this time towards the village.

So strange – walking in a familiar landscape so I was not surprised as each house and garden went by – but also had no idea of the wider context – where exactly were the shops? What was round the next corner? Again – just happening, noticing, no hurry.

And turning a corner, I came to the big car park and there was The Library! I was so excited. Once I had loved Libraries, spent hours in them, as a child discovering the wonders of reading. I remember many years ago when I came back on holiday from Boarding School, I would go to the Library where my sister worked – and I would sit for hours under her desk reading comics (not allowed at school) that she had saved for me – and collecting a pile of new books to read during the holidays.

I hadn't in fact been to a Library (other than the University one) for years, but I used to love to go to this Penmaenmawr Library to introduce my children to reading. Of course it really was different – they have computers in there now – and very few actual books. And of course I wasn't a member. And this was where I began to realise how much I was part of this community – so many people seemed to know me – I often did not know who they were – this thing of not recognising people took a while to get used to.

But everyone seemed to know what had happened to me – I met with so much kindness that day… and in the days to come.

They made me a member – gave me a card which I felt very proud of and left me to choose a book.

I have left a gap here on the page as I write this because – as I know now – choosing anything had become an almost impossible undertaking. Even now to choose a book in a shop or online is very hard. I cannot easily make my brain choose between things – and it was a shock to stand there and the sensation of this – I knew what I was meant to do but I couldn't do it.

So I just picked up two books that I liked the look of. I liked that they had nice pictures on the cover and they were big. I don't know what their titles were – I never read them – but enjoyed carrying them back home where they sat on the table and I just liked having library books. I know I went to the Library a lot then for a while – and sometimes got another book. They knew I didn't read them – they just let me come in – look, sit... so kind.

The next big adventure was going a bit further than the Library into the Village... I couldn't manage buying food yet (someone else seemed to provide that – not quite sure how now)... but I saw the café and went in – again – people knew me... so wonderful to sit there watching other people around me chatting. I think I sat there for hours drinking milky coffees.

All this was so simple – it was teaching me about small pleasures and the delights of little things – a cup of coffee, the warmth of the cup in my hands, the kindness of the smiles of people, the wonder that I can go out of my door and all these things are just there.

I was in pain – sometimes the headaches were dreadful. My whole body still ached and hurt – that phrase (why do I feel I have been run over by a steamroller) often in my head as I struggled – up or down stairs, to get in and out of bed, to walk back up the hill. But I did it – I had such an urge that I must push, follow what I had to do.

Isn't it strange that this first six months was in many ways a wonderful time? I was like a child – delighting in learning – feeling so cared for. Surrounded by all this beauty – my bedroom view which I had often barely glanced at before – in too much of a hurry to get on and do something or go somewhere.

And over the next month or so my brain was growing and growing, I was getting more confident – I was learning to manage myself – know my vulnerabilities. How far I could go and not go. How to know when I needed to stop and ask for help – I don't think I ever met with a rejection – I was, I suppose, a little old lady with a stick... I wonder if I was as kind to others as they had all been to me? I was learning (not without a lot of getting lost, exhausted and often distressed) how to get buses – go into shops and buy things – plan meals – do all the daily things that we have to do in life.

I went further on the Bus. I remembered the Conwy Bird Reserve which has always been one of my favourite places and one day managed to get the Bus there and (with some help) walk there along the river bank, and collapsed in their Café – so tired but thrilled. And just watched out of their big viewing windows. I couldn't use my binoculars – that was sad, but I just couldn't focus through them anymore.

And it was in the Reserve Café that the next exciting development occurred – and it had nothing to do with birds. They have a section for second hand books and toys and I saw some Jigsaws. I have always HATED Jigsaws, the most boring activity in the world, I thought (probably largely because I was 'no good' at them). But just as I wanted the piece of chocolate cake at the café I wanted a Jigsaw. And I bought one for £1 and proudly brought it home.

I think I enjoyed that process of doing that first Jigsaw as much as I had ever enjoyed anything! Very, very slowly finding a place for a piece. Before, I would have been impatient. Now I could take a few hours to think, to find where a piece fitted. Some days only a few would be placed. It was not the wanting to finish or see the completed picture but there was a pure joy in the process of searching and then finding and then searching. And when my son F came to visit, he sat with me and we did the Jigsaw together – so it grew a lot quicker then. Such fun, that sharing of the process. And for a while I did jigsaws – and somehow it was important – as if I was also building the jigsaw of my shattered brain.

Pain was my constant companion – and sometimes the sense of my head shifting inside and the ache at the back and stabbing burst of pain at the front were just there – at first I know I just wanted it to go away completely – going over that childhood rhyme in my head, 'rain, rain go away, come again another day' – and then we would all shout 'go away forever'. But of course it never did. And nor have the headaches. And I think the moment where they became somehow manageable was when I remembered that rhyme and, just like with rain, realised that if I just kept hoping it would go away, I would just keep myself discontented and unhappy. And perhaps that was a beginning part, too, of the process of accepting me the way I now was.

And as my brain shifted and opened I remembered the lines of a favourite song, Leonard Cohen's 'Anthem': 'That's where the light gets in'. I could FEEL in my head as new things came in – my brain is like a muscle – just like when you raise your arm slowly and notice what that is like you will notice the movement – the places where it is comfortable or uncomfortable – if you move your arm up and hold it in the air for a while you will notice the point where, if you hold it up long enough, it gets tired and you want to rest it. You will learn how long you can hold your arm in the air for! The brain is like that too. I felt the parts of my brain I could move a little more now, I could stretch my brain.

But my brain got tired very quickly. And that was what I had to learn. That I had to spot the tiredness – when I had done enough – even if that was only a short walk, or one conversation, or a few pieces of jigsaw, I began to learn when to stop and rest. And if I pushed too far through that, then my brain collapsed. I could feel that, the shutting down, a dull ache that is different to the headache – a nausea – and my eyes would become tired – I could hardly make myself see – it was an effort to make words. All I could do was rest – and, if I overdid it, rest for a few days.

And this does not change – indeed, we are all like that all the time – it is just that we have different levels of tolerance. I had to learn where mine were.

I was beginning to get a sense now that I was indeed on a journey. Those first weeks of many people coming, helping me and doing everyday survival tasks were passing. People had to go back into their own lives – workers assigned to me, I suppose to 'get me going', needed to go on to their next patients.

And oh, the weariness and difficulty of everyday tasks. Keeping yourself and your surroundings clean. Feeding yourself and all that entails. Buying food, putting it somewhere. Remembering where it was. Remembering how to prepare it… there are many stages to feeding ourselves! Keeping clothes clean and remembering what was dirty and what was not. And then, having worked out what needed doing and how to do it, I would take my attention off it for a while. Maybe I sat down for a rest, made a cup of tea, played a round of Patience… and then whatever it was I had remembered or decided to do would have completely disappeared from my memory. Just going upstairs for something, it was unlikely that by the time I was up the stairs I would know what it was I was there for. This means that doing anything takes ages and can be an exhausting and distressing process.

I am writing about this because managing these basic life tasks can be so terribly hard. And because I found that – for the most part – people simply do not understand that at all. The most common response to my sharing these difficulties has always tended to be an assumption that this is just the same as it is for everyone; we all have those 'senior moments' or sudden lapses in memory. But there is something about the quality of this loss with Brain Injury which has a very different quality – and also it happens, or happened to me, particularly in those first years, so frequently and so absolutely.

It made everything that bit more difficult – and, when going out, often frightening. Where am I? How did I get here? How do I get back? The added exhaustion of finally getting myself down to the village to buy milk and oats (main items of sustenance) and arriving in the shop with all knowledge of that gone. Complete blank. Make a list, people say. I made lists. Endless lists. However you have to remember 1) That you made the list. 2) To bring it with you. 3) To remember it is with you and look at it!!!!

And there were two things for me to do at those points – one would be to just collapse and cry and the other was to laugh. And I learned that the important thing when I noticed, was to praise myself for noticing, and have a strategy for what to do next.

My main strategy for these situations is to pause, deliberately smile, and if possible find somewhere to sit down.

I did a Breathing Space Meditation at those moments, adapted to suit me in those moments of early brain slipping – and still do.

BREATHING SPACE MEDITATION
Pause and say to myself:
What's going on for me right now. In my head and my body?
Just let yourself notice.
Tell yourself IT IS OK. You are OK.
Smile. Feel the smile. Feel the weight of your body sitting or standing here.
Follow your breathing In and Out… In and Out.
And coming out of the practice and looking around and noticing how you are Now.

Generally that will have calmed me – and with that I would often recall what I was there to do (this ONLY comes with allowing – NEVER with getting stuck TRYING to remember or FIND the information). Or I will have recalled there is a list and where I put it – or, if I still don't know why I am there, I can make a plan of what to do next and will have remembered that it is usually helpful to sit down and rest for a while and ideally find somewhere to have a cup of tea, maybe a cake. Going to a new shop or somewhere crowded is not a helpful thing to do – so there is a lot of learning and much of it is around the environment of the shopping and managing the almost inevitable slipping of memory.

And of course quite often I did not remember, so would come home and then realise no milk etc. And I learned too that the important thing then was to be kind to myself, not in any way criticise or blame myself, the situation or anyone else. This just brings more suffering and despair. I think I was learning to ACCEPT. To accept the way I was and also to be curious about it. I think my view of the whole thing as a journey was helpful here. And I spent a lot of my time writing in my journal, drawing how I saw the world.

And I knew two things – one, that I was different – that I did not live in the world I had been in before – I was surrounded by it but somehow not in it – I had walked through a Gate. I could see the Gate but not what was ahead.

As I looked back through the Gate I could see the old world – it seemed busy and crowded and noisy but when I stepped out of my house into it everything was changed – and I did not know my way around.

I can feel it now as I write – searching… searching for whatever it is that is lost now. And it is exhausting. And my mind is rearranged – I would pick my way then over the cracked mud of the Tsunami-buried streets – crawl down the ruined streets of memory. And somehow perhaps find something, maybe a house or room left standing, or hiding somewhere amid the changed landscape. There is a light – familiarity – little organised pockets of memory amid the rubble.

I heard how, after the Tsunami in Japan, whole streets were changed, roads clogged, buildings destroyed. You could not go from A to B because the pathways had gone.

And I have gradually learned to walk the pathways of my mind. To build new ways to get from A to B (if they are still there).

Later to build little islands in the sea of mud. And I would live for a while on one island, then another – never a whole world. That has never returned – the whole landscape of mind I had before.

And I can see now how clever – how inventive we are, how inventive I was. And it is a lonely journey because no one, not even the dear, dear people who supported me, can really know what it is like to be in that landscape. And I was glad of that, for them. And I was learning already, in my body, not in my head, that this was how it was and I had to learn my way around this landscape on my own.

We all long to help others by making things the same – helping them to return to how things were. Recovery is seen as getting back to how things were, for the most part.

That is familiar to me, in caring for a child who had so many operations, so much brain damage, so many life changing events. I had learned that you go day by day, it is no use wanting things to be different or railing against the past or future. Just needing to be with what unfolded now. And maybe too having been working as a Psychotherapist – again – to BE WITH people as they are now, in this moment. And could I do this now for myself? And in how I responded to all those around me – because they were struggling too.

We often want recovery to be making things better and the same because we cannot bear the sadness of the loss. And this is the human condition. Illness and injury and loss and abandonment come and go within the fabric of our lives.

And I had, too, my Mindfulness practice – curiosity rather than anxiety – acceptance through the curiosity – what's happening now?! – ability to notice and bring attention to the contact of my body, walking, sitting, lying and breathing. Just allowing whatever was here to be here – however it was.

Chapter 4: That's How the Light Gets in

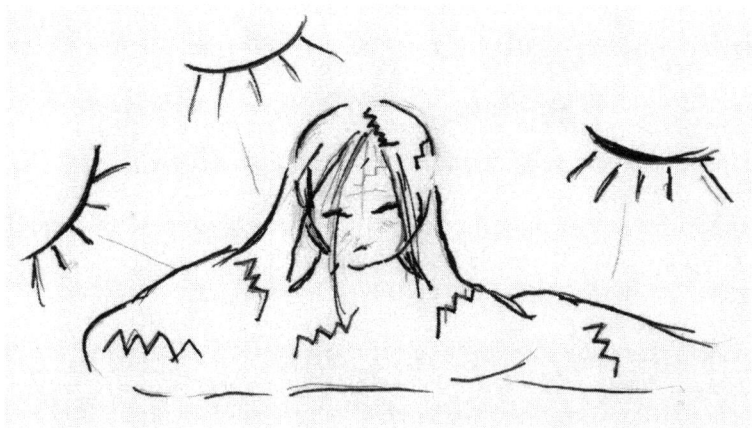

*'There is a crack, a crack in everything
That's how the light gets in.'*
(Leonard Cohen)

As the early weeks go by, patterns emerge – a wonderful lady called Tegwyn came to clean for me and collect shopping, and she was so good at helping me know what was needed and what to buy. I had been trying, I think, to see back, back into then to know what I needed to do now. And that didn't work. And now I gave up to that. I still spent a lot of time just propped up in my great bed looking out of the window – watching again in this moment the sea and sky change, moment by moment.

I am the same yet different. Some aspects of me seem to have dropped away completely and I am welcoming new aspects as they arise. We think we see, hear, know what is there. But we don't. We can only know this moment.

My house seemed strange – it was familiar but I no longer felt comfortable surrounded by so much colour, so many pictures and books. I didn't wear most of my clothes, they did not seem to belong to me. Cleaning my teeth in the morning I would see me in the mirror and feel again the shock of the stranger who was me. I often did not know who people were when I met them in the street, or when they first came to the house – did not recognise them – but I learned that if I stopped trying to work out who they were in my head but just experienced the feel of being with them, the sense of them, then I would know them. Though not necessarily their name.

Things around me still moved, objects that should stay still moving at the edge of my vision.

I was beginning to read… this was on my Kindle, such a wonderful device, I could make the letters huge and it was easy to hold. I could not manage books themselves; just holding them open seemed difficult. And interestingly, my taste in books had changed, I only wanted to read biographies – not stories.

The first book I read was Laurie Lee's *As I walked out one Midsummer Morning*. I wrote down the words *'it was one of those sudden, jerky advances in life, which, once made, closes the past for ever'*. And I wrote that in my journal – I spent a lot of time writing in journals – and I wrote *'oh the relief of that! Let the past as it unfolds moment by moment become sepia – old snapshots – captured but never kept because the memory changes – fades – embroiders – while the moment is clear – sharp – beautiful in its sometimes terrible strength because it is, and it can never be truly captured.'*

Family, friends, come and go. We carry on in some ways as normal. All my family are here one day and we have, just as we always have had, an evening meal – all sitting together. In many ways it was lovely – but I wrote in my journal, *'I found our family meal difficult last night. I felt so disconnected from everyone – as if I almost wasn't there. Everyone seems to shout – there is a lot of laughter, jokes. I don't like jokes, I realise I don't understand what is going on. I want us to just sit together in silence, or to play a game. I am always wanting now to play a game together. I am not sure why. I don't know how to be. It is upsetting to feel so separate, so cut off. These are my beloved children. I don't seem to be able to respond within conversations so I sit quiet. What has happened to me. What is going to happen. I don't tell them because I don't quite understand and also I don't want them to worry about me any more than they already do. We were all having to get to know me again. I want the same. And so I wasn't the same mother. How sad is that'*.

This of course became a long journey, and one which, years later, in many ways we are all still on. I don't think I realised I had a Brain Injury then – but the impact is huge and it is huge for family members. They had me back but I was not the same. And we all had to learn how to be with that. These were early days.

Friends were visiting a lot now too – other family talking on the phone. My head exhausted, my brain constantly 'slipping', that now-familiar sense of pressure in my head and an inability to remember what just happened – to 'grasp' things. I often felt 'fizzing or lightning' shock-type sensations in my brain… to start with I found that alarming but I am used to it now. I think it happens more when I am tired. People kept saying 'you are just the same as you were', wanting to reassure me. How isolated that made me feel, but at this point I really began to try and open to compassion, for me and for others,

I must keep hold of that. This is tough for everyone. No one really knows what to say. It was a relief one morning when Tegwyn came to clean and said 'you don't look as good as last week'.

I suppose I was getting used to the territory of me now. Daily walks, the business of life, reading, listening to the radio, jigsaws. I found a half finished cushion cover to embroider, there was a simple picture of a tree to set the stitches around… and I found an old rainbow wool jumper I had knitted for my daughter. And I had an image of it unravelling. And I thought this is me. This is how I am. I am a brightly coloured rainbow jumper but someone unravelled it. And then if I knitted it again it would look the same on the surface but of course it would be different, subtle different placing of sequences of colour.

It was still a colourful functional jumper. I remember the power of that for me. I am different but I am still a me and a functional person. I will live in the world as I am now. I wrote that in big letters. I will live in the world as I am now. And that meant not regretting, not wanting anything to be different. I would feel the sadness of the loss, the excitement of achieving new things or relearning. Around then I began to be able to do more of my Mindfulness Practices and as I sat, for perhaps as long as 20 minutes now, breathing, I also intentionally brought in Acceptance. Acceptance of myself and of how everything around me is. And compassion. Compassion for myself in this great change, and for all those others, particularly my family, who are having to come on this often difficult journey with me.

And there was more purpose now in my outings. I went to Llandudno with the intention of finding a Wedding Tapestry or Embroidery set so that I could sit and sew and also make a gift for my daughter D and her fiancé C, who were getting married next year.

And I found one – in an excellent shop I had only just discovered – just perfect – lovely colours and I could change some of the details to fit for D and C. And I knew how to do this – this was something from my past, childhood – sewing. And knitting too, and none of these old skills seemed to be lost.

And this turned into a momentous day. I had my Tapestry set. And somehow that had given me the confidence to go into another shop, and I went into Waterstones Book Shop. All those books, colours. I had looked in there earlier on when in Llandudno because it was one of my favourite places to go. But at that time I could not tolerate being there, the stacked books seemed to fall forwards onto me from the shelves, the colours moving, everything in motion, and I had left, shaken, on that visit. But on this day the movement was not enough to send me out – it was still there – but I was getting used to these perceptual shifts now. I was not so overwhelmed by them. And I went up to the Café and ordered a coffee. I remember sitting there. So pleased to be back in that environment. Feeling the familiarity of it. This is home!

I knew not to try to look at the books, usually I would buy some. I would get lost, I knew in looking and trying to make a choice. But as I sat there I could see nearest to me some shelves of Poetry Books. And a name stood out for me, Wendy Cope. I liked her poems and I had met her some time ago when we were staying in the same place, and I thought – I am meant to look at that book. And I went and got it and brought it back to the table. And it was *A Poem a Day*, edited by Nicholas Albery with a foreword by Wendy Cope. And it felt magical, it was just the right thing for me. A poem a day and I could see many were old friends. And I bought it. And out of all the many things I did, discovered, people brought for me, this book has been perhaps the most important of my whole journey of recovery.

I even felt confident finding the Bus stop and coming home that day. Something had shifted in my recovery.

These things, particularly the Tapestry and the Book of Poems, were things from my past, they had nothing to do with my immediate life before but they connected me to old knowledge, the me that seemed to have gone. On that journey home, walking up the hill from the bus stop, more adept now with my stick, sitting in bed and looking out again over the sea, the so familiar and yet completely different and new view, I knew that I was no longer in that old pre-haemorrhage world, I was on a bridge. I had gone through the Gate and was walking slowly along a narrow bridge, high above the sea. It was a Rope bridge, wobbly, high, fragile, and I could not turn around, the end was too far away to see. I could only be in this moment, with this step. The old world was behind me. And beyond the Gate.

I could only be in each moment, each event and whatever I am doing – nothing is very planned or structured, I just let whatever is here be here. Sit and do a jigsaw, go for a walk, get on the bus and see where I get off. So many friends visiting, colleagues coming to take me out to shop for food, or buying food for me. Being taught how to do a Tesco shop online – although I am still a long way from being able to do all that – turning on the computer, logging on… but it will come. Life, even life after brain haemorrhage, often moves in phases. I am immersed in the poems, reading them over and over again.

That brought home to me the loneliness of recovery and also the contact that comes from the practices, connection with the breath, and the connection and contact from all my visitors, and how I never felt alone. Even in hospital, when I was alone and in pain, I had the memory of my children's hands, could feel the weight of them on mine even when they were not there. And the softness of the contact of the sheet that my hands were resting on. And realised that I had been doing a Loving Kindness meditation then, noticing the contact, feeling the love and compassion of others. These are the things that are getting me through, through the dark, alone, bewildered and painful times.

And a miracle happened, or so it seemed to me. Here I was unable to remember anything much, never mind what day it was, what happened yesterday, what I might have said to someone on the phone this morning, what was on the radio half an hour ago. Everything seemed to slip away, so that there was only this moment. Yet I found I could learn poems by heart. It was easy, if I liked one somehow it felt as if I absorbed it – and then I had them with me everywhere, whenever I wanted them. I became hungry, hungry to learn, take in, poems. And this one, *All you who sleep alone...* was the first one I learned – it is still here six years later. I began to go to Llandudno, learn to go on my computer again so that I could buy books of poems from Amazon, and download onto my Kindle. I could feel my brain working, like a rusty tool, and poems were oiling it all, making my brain more fluid.

And a round of busyness began and I made the journey on my own, on the train up to Liverpool to Walton Outpatients – my first hospital visit on my own since the Haemorrhage. Taking time to map out the journey, getting on trains, changing trains. I learned that I needed a list of stations I needed to change at – but that was all I could remember anyway. I just had to deal with each bit of the journey as it happened. Get off here. Find a sign to the next station – often I had to ask because the lists were confusing – but there are always people to help. Up that escalator. Ask someone. Down that passage. Ask someone... just taking each bit at a time.

It was no good trying to hold the whole journey in mind, it would all just slip and I would be quite disorientated. And getting out at Fazakerly which is five minutes from the hospital and walking with my stick down icy pavements. The hardest bit was crossing the road. Two wide streams of traffic and lots of flashing coloured lights. I took a long time. Stopped in the island in the middle and watched what others did until I was quite sure. Then all the way back again – three hours there and three hours back. But I had no sense of time – there was no such thing as a long time or a short time, just now. I enjoyed being on the trains and the challenge, though also quite a lot of anxiety about getting lost, of finding my way to change trains.

I was so exhausted when I got home and so pleased. This was a huge step forward, but also another reminder of how different I was, how different the world about me was. It took me days to recover, the headaches blinding, my body aching, hard to move. I could not even read my poems or listen to the radio; everything had to stop so I could recover. My brain could not take anything more in. Another learning. Though I had to do this lots more times before I finally remembered it was not a good idea, I needed to put limits on what I did.

And suddenly things moved quickly – there was a plan for me to go on the train down to Brighton to stay with D and C for a few days. I could travel,

I had been going out to Llandudno, I had been into cafés. It would be good for me. I could get one train all the way to Euston and C would meet me there and take me on down to Brighton. I knew Brighton well, I knew the journey well, what could the problem be? What could go wrong? I was fearful and excited. Someone must have bought my tickets... I had to pack.

Packing can be difficult at the best of times – to take just enough, not too much and the right things... we have all been there. Generally I was quite good at packing. And if I didn't have what I wanted, I could buy something new – this was one of the joys of going to Brighton – or had been. I did pack – but learned the utter exhaustion that can come from making choices – I didn't seem to be able to make choices at all easily any more. I might put one item of clothing in the bag and then speak to someone and have forgotten what I had already packed – K helped and F took me to the station... and I was on my own all the way to Euston and meeting C. This was the woman who had hitchhiked over many countries on her own – thought of herself as a seasoned traveller, first travelled alone from London to Wales to a new school aged seven. Now I needed babysitting!

But it was easy. I loved just sitting and looking out of the window, and getting out at Euston, the excitement of arriving. C was waiting for me, and I was glad that he was there because again this familiar place looked different, the noise level was almost unbearable, all the posters and screens were wavering and moving, everything seemed to scream at me. I was bumping into people to start with – they all moved so much faster than I was. I put my head down, let myself be led – escalators – undergrounds – Victoria – a crowded commuter train. In and out of gates, through tunnels – Brighton Station. It was the sudden babble of noise and so many people all around me – something else to get used to.

Neuro Notes 1: Early Recovery

Some changes caused by a stroke or brain injury will be obvious straight away. Others may take longer to show up.

The person may not fully understand what has happened. They may feel confused, upset and worried.

The person is likely to feel unwell at first – dizziness, muscle pain and headaches are very common. They may be extremely tired and need to sleep and rest a lot. Peace and quiet is important.

Doing things will be very tiring. The person may not be able to do many things, or to keep going for very long. It is often helpful to ask the person to make simple choices about what they need and want.

Difficulties will improve, but it can be hard to predict how much. This uncertainty can be unsettling. Early recovery needs to be taken one day at a time.

Physical changes, such as difficulty with walking or speech, may improve faster than changes in memory or emotion or behaviour.

An injury to the brain slows it down. It cannot cope with as much, or work as fast as it did. Everything may seem overwhelming or confusing.

A person with a stroke or brain injury is likely to have problems with concentration, memory, planning and organisation.

The person may become more aware of their difficulties as they begin to do more. These discoveries can be very upsetting. Other people take longer to recognise their difficulties, and this is not at all unusual.

The person may not remember how to do things – or realise what needs to be done. They may need prompting and reminding, help with breaking tasks down into smaller steps, and doing one at a time.

The person may feel anxious about trying to do things, and may need patience, reassurance and encouragement to re-build their confidence.

The person may behave differently, or be more difficult to get along with. These changes can be distressing for everyone involved.

Part 2: Cannot Go That Way Again

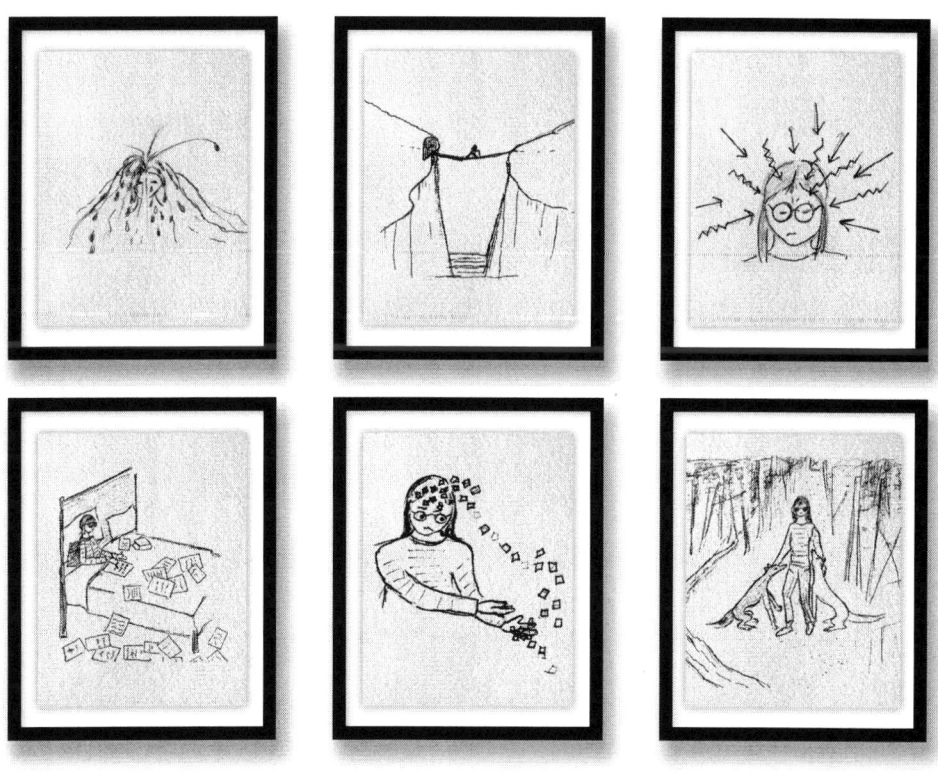

Chapter 5: Over the Rope Bridge

And as the evening twilight fades away, the sky is filled with stars invisible by day.

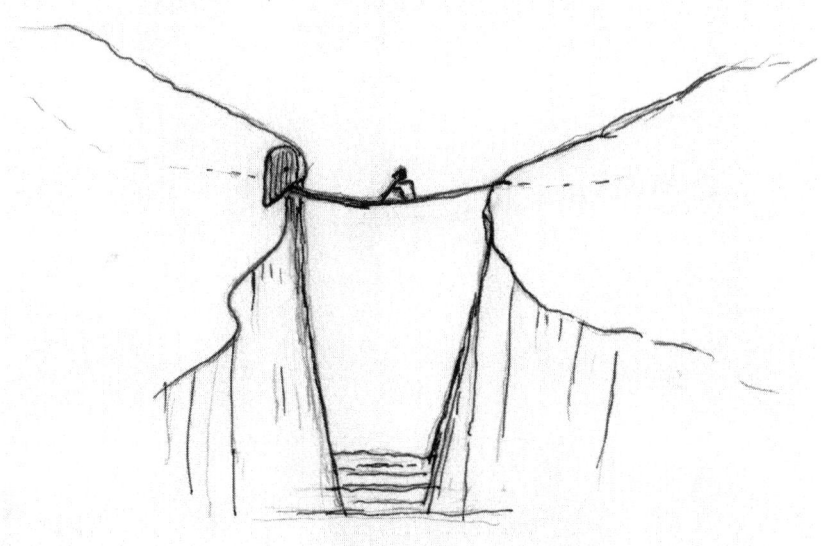

I am in a different land – I realise here in this familiar place that I cannot go back – I am changed – everything around me is changed – I can only go on. Behind me the Rope Bridge I have just stepped off hangs between my past and present over a deep ravine and the oceans of the world. I am on a parallel path – it is completely alone – no one else is there. And as I walk, from time to time I find myself in these sudden pockets of noise and activity – like travelling through the desert and arriving at a populated oasis – people eating, drinking, celebrating. And I am just passing through. Like a ghost – I am not really there. But I can enjoy watching them, like in an Art Gallery or watching a play. I talk with them – but it is not me – communication is strange – as if through an interpreter.

We get a taxi up the hill and to the haven of their flat and D is waiting for me. Such a relief to be there. So wonderful to be with my daughter. Familiar, familiar amid the unfamiliarity – even here things looking different. Just finding my way around, getting in and out of bed, washing and cleaning teeth and all those daily things that need a lot more conscious attention than we would usually give them. We do so many things automatically – I could feel as if a day's work was done by the time I was finally up, dressed, breakfasted and ready to go anywhere!

The plan was to spend three days together, walk in the Lanes, choose a Wedding Dress for D and do other Wedding related shopping – meet with friends and have meals out. All the normal things you do. I start off well; to some extent I have adapted to the crowds of people and the sense of the colours and sides of buildings shifting and moving in my peripheral vision. I expect this now so I am adjusting to my new reality, and I begin to relearn how to pace my walking and enjoy looking in the windows, stopping for Coffees and Croissants, making plans together, as we always had.

I find it helps me to deliberately bring my attention to just what is happening in this moment, not letting my mind go into worrying about crashing or how things will be later. I let the activity of movement that is constantly there at the edge of my vision just be there. Saying over and over to myself 'it is OK, just how I am now'. Then I could stay with what was in front of me, the next step, or what someone was saying to me or what we were looking at now in this shop. It helped that D and I had often shopped here before; I found the familiarity soothing even though the unfamiliarity of the movement and noise was distressing.

We went to a lovely Vintage Shop and looked at Wedding Dresses, talking, planning, choosing and D being measured. I remember I was trying to be as I would have been – I knew that I would have contributed more – had ideas – made suggestions. Would have enjoyed it all more. I didn't feel as if I was being particularly helpful and began to feel the fatigue building and fighting it, 'we are only at the beginning, too much to do, don't crash, don't crash'. It was all the stimulus around me and also making decisions – giving my opinion – I think, rather than the actual walking, that I found tiring, and by the time we have made decisions in the Sewing Machine Shop too I am exhausted.

But I am not doing too badly – I am functioning, making decisions, remembering things. But D tells me that I am 'still forgetting things' – and I realise that a lot of what I am recalling is different to what we actually did – things have dropped away – I often remember when reminded, sometimes not – and for the first time I become aware that I repeat things a lot. I remember feeling shocked and embarrassed as I realised that – and this became a familiar pattern – I know now that I forget – say things again and again, change the story, again and again, block out things that happen – rearrange things in my head. I hated this at first, I felt so out of control and I could not trust myself – is what I remember, what happened? Is what I am saying right or am I muddling it up? Does what I say make sense? What will people think of me?... for the first time since the haemorrhage, as I came into more contact with others, I began to feel anxious, not so much about my ability in the environment, though that was there, but about how I was seen, about my impact on others.

We went out for a meal with some of D and C's friends, some of whom I knew… to a lovely Brighton restaurant called Mange Tout, and that was familiar as we had been there together before. There seemed to be so many people there and the tables seemed close together – the walls moving and falling in on me – choices about food – I could not focus in and hear what was being said to me – music, a babble of talk and laughter, bright lights, choices, questions, I remember what became a familiar sensation of closing down, tightness in my jaw, it was hard to speak – because I could not hear what was being said to me, I felt out of control and out of contact and I was hoping I looked normal, no one would notice. And probably they didn't, I struggled to eat, to focus on the food, battered by all the movement around me. The movement and noise making me separate, dizzy.

I rather lost my confidence about being with people at that time, though we met other friends, and even danced the next day! I think I could do that because we went to a Tea Dance and I was dancing a Waltz – another thing I learnt to do very young. In my body, old learning, none of the problems of trying to remember recent learning in my head. The setting for the tea dance, the age of most of the people there, the 1950s décor, all familiar to me. The noise level much lower than in so many places and so although still very aware of it I was not overwhelmed as I had been in other places. So interesting how these early learnings and memories have stayed but things that are more recent seem to have gone or are more vulnerable to being changed – reinvented. I supposed that was what I was doing, reinventing myself. Perhaps we have to do that. It is hard to be without an identity – to some extent we create and recreate the person we are as we grow and in different situations… I was completely recreating myself – finding out who and what I was moment by moment, much of what I had trusted and known about myself suddenly untrustworthy, could not be reached.

Remembering again Laurie Lee's words in *As I Walked Out One Midsummer Morning*:

'It was one of those sudden, jerky advances in life which, once made, changes the past forever.'

I could not go back. The past was closed. I could never be the same again – and strangely, I didn't really want to be – though I knew that mostly, other people were expecting that to happen. Generally when we suffer severe illness or an accident we either die, or become an invalid and retire from work, or come back and carry on as before. And of course, that is not how it is with a brain injury. You come back different to before. No one is prepared for it, least of all you.

The Brighton visit was so many things; wonderful, fun, enjoyable – empowering, so much I can do, remember, and I do have skills. Though many of them may not be particularly relevant to getting back to work as a psychotherapist and mindfulness trainer! Or perhaps they were. Dancing, sewing, tapestry, painting, learning poems, watching nature, the sea, the sky. These were the foundations of my learning and they were returning now.

The seeds of difficulties I was to encounter in returning to my world, life, family and work were there in that early Brighton visit.

How I was in myself and with others, how they perceived me. I have always been confident socially, able to converse – remember details about people – demonstrate interest in them. One of my particular interests and perhaps talents has been the perceptual – colours – shapes – enjoyment of art galleries – designing, creating, reading, with going on visits to look at things – shopping. Enjoying seeing what is there, what I like, knowing what others would like and what would suit them, able to make quick choices – let's get that for… for Christmas – oh – lets have that theme for the tree, the house it will fit with… That jumper would suit… It will go with… And make quick decisions to buy. What paintings, furnishings, draperies would go somewhere – a new wardrobe theme for the Autumn.

And I was planning for not just one but two weddings. My daughter getting married next July and my son in September. And there were stories – how many stories I have read and always remembered would link to themes – to colour combinations – to tell the story of lives. How busy and inventive my brain was.

I didn't know how important all that was until I lost it. And in Brighton on that visit, that loss was marked. I was interested in buying the wedding dress and all the bits and pieces that go with it but didn't have the energy or mental focus to maintain an active enthusiasm as I would have. My ability to stay in the story, to maintain attention and interest, seemed so diminished, I felt diminished.

Now I was concerned, and a little frightened – how would things be? How could I go back to work? More importantly, how will I be at the weddings? Such are the priorities of life. Much of my attention, I realise now, was focused on getting back to work and D's wedding.

So back to the journey home from Brighton. I had gained confidence, things still moved and closed in on me from my peripheral vision. I had begun to accept that as not a pleasant experience, but something that was there. I was finding a way to ground, that was, to firmly feel my feet on the ground and my body standing or sitting, focus in and breathe, at the same time as being aware of and allowing the chaos and movement that might be around me. Getting out of the train at Victoria, a mass of bustling people, noise, lights. I found a bench and sat for a while, forgetting about time (not difficult as I didn't have much of a sense of time anyway) and allowing the mind to settle. And looked around.

And Victoria station is another familiar place, and although much changed, the shape of where the platforms are, the ticket office, the entrance to the Underground were all the same as years ago. And I went through familiar motions of going through the barricades, down the escalators, following just the one sign – Euston. And I got the right train. And I have wondered about that, about the brain, about familiarity from childhood and familiarity from later in life.

And, unlike before when I loved to explore new places, since the Haemorrhage I have been most happy and settled in familiar surroundings, even if, as in the case of this visit to Brighton, they were familiar long ago. This theory is borne out I think in that the two biggest of my 'brain crashes' have occurred when changing trains and in Birmingham New Street station. Partly because it did not exist when I was a child, and if it did I never went there – and also because it is a nightmare of a station anyway!

And I had achieved a journey – and learnt so much, some painful, some joyful – and that I still had what it takes to find my way through! And, even more important, we had got the Dress, which after all is what I had gone to do. And there is comfort too, I think, in these normal rituals of human lives – weddings, ceremonies, traditions. I was still here.

I was learning the 'New Normal'. Others look for us to return to being as before, to be 'the same' as them. But the widened perception of brain injury, the different ways of pacing, noticing and being in the world, is simply a new normal. It is a development of a capacity to function. The old self belongs to before.

Chapter 6: Leave Everything You Know Behind

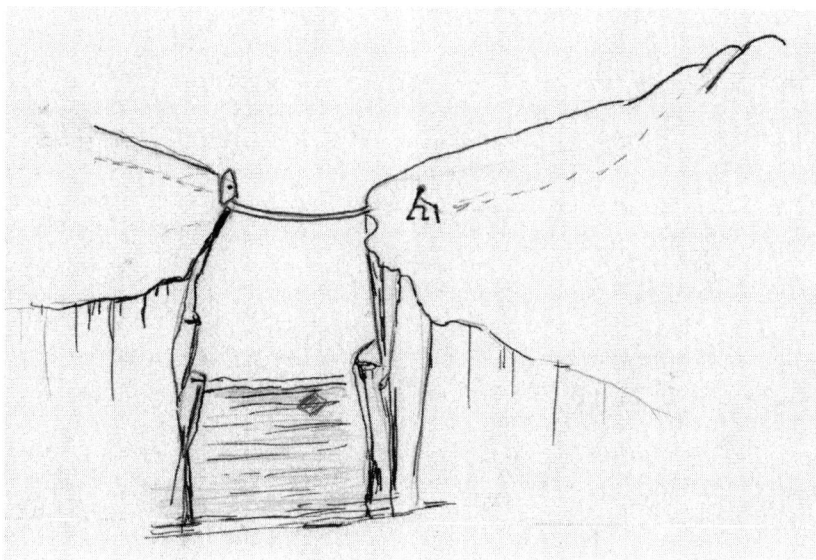

Effort of getting out and about

By the end of September I am doing so much more. I write in my diary, 'it is hard work, this recovery'. I can manage to shop for food, make my meals, go out on the bus now, but it all takes such a long time and such a lot of effort. I do not seem to have the sense of time I had before either – so I often mis-time things… it is another level of awareness – what time of day it is, how long it will take to get somewhere – what day it might be – are the shops actually open?

I can manage the walk to the shops, and now even to the bus most days… but each activity involves such effort. Just looking at the shelf in the supermarket – the whole business of deciding what I need… remembering it, remembering to take a list – to look at the list. And then when I get it home it all has to be put somewhere. It is all so confusing and tiring I find it difficult to explain – each excursion is rather like planning and booking a holiday. Nothing seems automatic, it must all be done as if for the first time, over and over again.

Some days my brain would just crash. I could arrive in the village and have no idea what I was doing, where I was going or even how I got there. At first that was frightening but then I learnt to stop, to just sit on the bench by the Bus Stop. Just notice my feet on the ground, the contact of my body with the bench, and watch the movement of my breath… this breath all the way in… this breath all the way out. And to trust, remind myself this had happened before, I will know in a moment. Sometimes I would just go back home. Back to the safety and security of my bedroom and my view.

I spent much of my time, though, back lying on my wonderful bed, a refuge. And such a relief: every movement of my body could seem an effort. Sometimes I could not even remember how to get out of bed – or then how to get from one place to another – I would have to sit and wait for it to come back to me. No forcing. And it could be frightening, but I had learned to let go when that happened. This was another place where my Mindfulness Practice was so helpful and supportive, as at the Bus Stop bench.

GROUNDED BREATHING PRACTICE
Notice the contact of my body with the sheets
Feel the weight of my body against the bed – supported
Bring my attention to the movement of the in breath and the out breath
Feeling the sensation of the breath in the nostrils and the mouth
The rise and fall of the belly with the breath
Letting go of any tension
Dropping into just lying there breathing
And noticing any thoughts
Seeing if I could just allow them to pass
Not getting caught up in worries and thoughts
But just resting there, breathing in and out
For a few moments

And then I would look out of my wonderful window… aware always of how lucky I was to have this view, seeing the clouds moving over the sky and the sea, the birds too, flying past. And it helped me to stay in THIS moment, to not get caught up in my thoughts and worries and fears as we so easily do. To remind myself that these moments of exhaustion, sometimes despair, will also pass.

It was hard work, this thing called Recovery. Sometimes just to move, to get up, to wash took such concentration. Each movement had to be thought of, noticed… How my body hurt… how hard it was sometimes even to lift an arm… the pain and strange movements so often in my head. But also the places where I felt comfortable, perhaps warm… the pleasant feel of soft fabrics, the comfortable bed or chair.

I decided I needed to try and do some stretching exercises to loosen a little – just pushing at the edges of stretching. I found that anything that involved bending my head or neck was unpleasant – going gently… and bringing Compassion to myself, to my body. My whole body felt stiff… some parts, like my right arm and right foot, seemed harder to move. Even lifting my fingers could be an effort! How come a brain injury can have such a strong effect on the rest of the body?

Each day I tried to have a walk; some days it felt easier and then I might go off on the bus. But it all took a lot of effort. By the time I was up, dressed and had what I needed, I felt as if a day of work had gone by, and was exhausted.

Nevertheless usually I would start out. There was a determination – it almost felt beyond my will, that somewhere deep inside I knew I had to push to do this – to recover, however hard it was. Somehow it felt as necessary as food and water.

Each movement required a concentration of my mind – this step – now this step – and decisions, there are so many decisions we make out of awareness… to decide to get up, to get down from the bed or up from the chair, stand up, get food and drink, go out – with all that involves – you need a key, some money, appropriate clothing. All previously automatic decisions now thought of in so much more detail. So by the time I have got anywhere I have already run a marathon!

I found it was a lonely process and that no one really seemed to understand the effort I had to put in. And I began to feel what was to become a familiar loneliness… so often people would say – oh yes, we all feel like that sometimes… or at the end of the week… and I would think – no you don't… I have never experienced this before. I thought of a film with the title 'The Loneliness of the Long Distance Runner'. That was me.

First Christmas

It is late in December now. There is snow all around – perhaps turning to ice – throwing up uncertainty about whether our Christmas plans will happen. I am so TIRED and have been having increasingly strong headaches – woke at 4.25am with bad head – whole head throbbing with pain. Asking am I doing too much – what IS too much. I liked the days when there was no DOING stretching out around me – just Being – like a wonderfully soft duvet. But I also feel this urge – to stretch myself – my brain. Somehow I know that I have to keep going – push through this. Not sure why or what for – but a physical and mental need almost.

But the last few weeks have been so busy, taking a train to Crewe for a Mindfulness Teachers meeting – and such joy in contact with friends but also this terrible loss – because I am not the same – no one will say so – they say things like you're doing so well, great you are better now. Whatever that means. Am I better? Well, up and about – but I am very different. I found that saying to someone – what seemed so obvious and simple to me – well, yes I am much better than I was when I was in hospital and I can do a lot more – but that is my body – it gets very tired – so, so tired, and that is different – but what you don't see is that my internal experience is often so hard and unseen – except noticed by others if I stumble or go the wrong way – turn up late, don't know what we are talking about.

In a discussion there is huge effort involved in following the conversation – it feels rather like trying to lift and then hold a heavy boulder – if I let my attention stray I know it will all roll away and I will not remember any of it.

I find it hard to follow discussions – everyone seems to jump around and go so fast – I find it hard to interpret other facial expressions – so a sense of unease as not sure how they are responding to me. I have to think and concentrate very hard to form words and sentences to communicate what I want to say. When we go to lunch – or other rooms in the house; we go in and out of doors and along corridors – that now familiar sense of walls falling in on me. I hate going into toilets – fear always there, will I ever find my way out again?

This difficulty with Toilets has remained – I feel more secure now because I know from experience that I will get out and I will get back to wherever I came from. But toilets are necessarily often down stairs or in corridors or dark, out of the way places. You are supposed to lock yourself in them. Then you have to find your way back.

Even here, in the Retreat Centre that was vaguely familiar to me, with a group of caring friends and colleagues – over and over again I would get lost – there was no recall of which way I went before. Even now, I felt the sense of confusion and an almost physical aching in my head as I tried to remember the way – this may sound strange, but some doors (particularly in modern buildings – and in toilets) do not look particularly like doors. I would stand, and GROUND – feet on the floor… breathe… do not engage with the panicky thoughts – and my best strategy was to feel the walls for the door – and somehow that helped – although it could take a while. I remember when I realised I could do that – almost disconnect the trying to think bit of my brain, then I calmed – and trusted.

All this was going on as I did what everyone else did, talking – mostly I think – as if I was the same as before – but all the time I was an imposter. Really, I think as I write this, it was that thing of doing everything as if for the first time… and I so wanted to share that – but people mostly will not hear. They say – oh, we all experience that sometimes... NO THEY DON'T. Perhaps what is important here is again noting how much attention it takes for me to maintain an activity – and the toll that it takes.

I found it so strange that people, friends and colleagues, so often said – you are just the same. I found that so strange – I presumed they meant it, why would they lie, but also I found it very upsetting because there was no doubt at all for me that I was different, and to have that denied felt discounting, as if I was just making a fuss, nothing much had happened to me at all. And then my doubts would set in, am I making a fuss, could I do, see things better if I tried hard enough.

But I got used to this, realised it was just another part of having a Brain Injury, that it is difficult for other people perhaps to see the difficulties that are there – they want to see the positives – what is the same.

Nothing inside me was the same. I pause as I write that: is that true? Yes, yes, how can anything be the same because I am not the same person. And I realised how difficult that must be for others, perhaps it is scary, I don't know. And I stopped asking those questions, went along to some extent with the charade, and I felt good about that because it allowed me to stay close and connected to them. And eventually a wonderful group of my closest friends and colleagues did see – and being accepted just as I now am was the most healing thing I have experienced – I am so grateful to them all.

But now we were coming up to Christmas – always my favourite time of year. My first Christmas as this me.

This Christmas has a traditional feel – it is cold and snowy – the wheels of Christmas skidding on the icy roads... the frozen world of the birds in the back garden – song thrushes searching for food.

The heating has been off for two days – roads impassable – shops laid siege to. D and C are driving up over the snowy roads. It is exciting.

I like the sharpness of it all – even the cold – the beauty of snow and the blanket of quietness that it brings. Perhaps because my world seemed to have become often so loud and bright with unfiltered sound and lights since the brain haemorrhage... the stillness and peace was welcome.

Leave everything you know behind

Christmas is passing now – and somehow it feels as though it was a bridge from the Haemorrhage and recovering to a different level of recovery – what will this new year bring? On New Year's Eve at 12.00 we went out to the field behind where I live. D, C and me – the snow was luminous... a magical blue coloured moon – almost full I think… sending a bright light down over the snow. We all put our own interpretations on these sort of experiences of course – but for me in that moment, standing there in the mix of darkness and light and the movement from one year to the next, I remember I realised both how much I seemed to have lost, and also that I had to go forward now. This is a familiar New Year realisation, often with resolutions – but this year I was going forward as a different person – with changed abilities which I hardly yet knew about – and it felt daunting – and also… I made a choice that I would go and explore how I was in my life – with the changes I hardly knew yet – and it felt exciting – this was the new journey I had thought I might make to all my planned travelling destinations – I couldn't travel now – but I could travel inside.

When the Heart

When the heart
Is cut or bruised or broken
Do not clutch it
Let the wound lie open
Let the wind from the good old sea blow in
And bathe the wound with salt
And let it sting
Let a stray dog lick it
Let a small bird put its head inside the hole and sing
A simple song – like a tiny bell
And let it ring.
(Michael Leunig)

But as everyone left and went into their lives it is not so easy. My body seems to ache less but I am more and more aware of my mind… my brain…

There was a more or less constant ache and slipping in my head, hard to describe it but I cannot grasp – stay with things… the thought streams… memories… constantly trying to remember what I have just done – thought. Those incidents we all have of maybe going upstairs and then not remembering what we went up for – for me this had become almost constant – and I could get caught in the trying to grasp something – but it would slip away again. Sometimes to get from the bed to downstairs took forever, where was I going, up or down… I am down now, why, what was I going to do? I'd better go upstairs again; maybe I was going to clean my teeth or something.

There was no structure to my day, because I didn't know where I was in it, there was no time, just day and night – and so I took refuge in my safe activities… at that time playing endless games of Patience – without any aim, just watch each card, this card, this card, and sewing… and reading and learning Poems.

One morning when I woke, I wrote in my diary 'Leave everything you know behind'.

Such a relief, and then I could rest. It felt as though my mind was in need of activity – but other than structured repetitive activity I just didn't seem to be able to engage in it. Or I would just go back to my refuge of my bed and my view and just watch the constant change of the sea, the clouds, the weather, the birds. And it is as tiring as running up a mountain – and I realise I am much more emotional about it all than I was.

There is nowhere to escape to. Trying to work things out in my head, I feel pins and needles – muddle – things come and slip away in moments. I see I wrote in my journal 'There is nothing here… and too much here – too much noise – too much to see – no respite – no respite from being in my head… from being me – only I am not me'. I felt so disconnected and alone. When other people were there I think I had a sense of my identity… them and me… but on my own, in those early months, I was anchorless. Strangely, sometimes the pain was helpful – pain is grounding, I knew I was in pain. And sometimes it's as if I was still on my raft only now it was full of all my possessions and I had been pushed out to sea. I am a long way from anywhere. A long way from recovery. Whatever that is.

And those moments passed, as all moments do. This knowledge came from my Mindfulness Practice and again I was so grateful for it. The idea that everything passes – the constant reminders of this which I had from watching the sky and sea and birds and now too the season changes… all things pass… and if I just stay remembering and accepting that… not wanting things to be as they were or different to how they are in my brain… then it all becomes so much easier.

And actually, despite the discomfort and frequent pain, I am happy. I can learn to see this as an adventure – I am travelling a different territory to what was planned. I would let go of the ghosts of the past and step out into this new adventure. And I realised that it was going to be hard work. And strangely that too was helpful. It gave me a purpose.

Chapter 7: The Way Lies over the Mountains

Heading Home

*Over mountains,
a cloak of rolling clouds
for the noble standing
of the Nantlle kings.*

*At their feet,
the silken surface of lake,
with ripples spreading
like drops of kindness
from the heart
of the lovely Baladeulyn queen.*

*And in the wide clear openness above,
a lone circling buzzard –
calling.*

*We hold freeze framed,
these sights and sounds,
a teaching in the body mind.
Etching in us, intent –
to come back.*
(Trish Bartley, 2010)

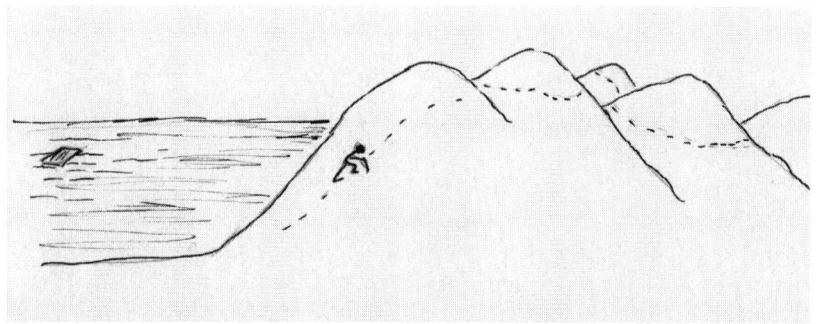

As I look back now on that time, the determination with which I stepped out and climbed the foothills and the peaks, I see more clearly how I was, without realising it, building the foundations of how we are in our bodies in the world.

We come from our experience of Thoughts and Feelings and usually we dance between the two, some lean more towards Thinking... Knowledge as a way of understanding, and others more towards sensation – perception – emotions. And of course we need both, both inform the other.

I can see how I unconsciously was trying to find ways to mend my shattered brain, and how these activities I was instinctively drawn towards were helping in this task.

Reading and memorising poems, sketching and painting, meditating, walking, these were all drawn from my need for sensations, feelings, reflection.
I understood myself from how I was Being, was experiencing my life – mapped it all out in pictures – found it in poems – in walking by the sea and under the trees. Here I was fully myself...

'Time present and time past. Are both perhaps present in time future.'
(T.S. Eliot *Burnt Norton*, from *Four Quartets*)

But these did not help me to function in the everyday world where I needed to feed myself, to keep the house clean, to get from A to B and to think, to plan, to organise. What I had taken for granted, that ability to write a list and to use it, to know what time of year and what day it was without effort. Just to remember.

I see now as I look back what I did not see then. How strong I was in this Being and how I was struggling with Doing... activities – with accessing my thinking and organising mind. I could reflect; indeed, I was so much closer to a world of sensation and present moment awareness. As I sat up in my bed and gazed from hour to hour, sometimes for days, out over the ocean, I sometimes felt the walls and window dissolve between me and the sea. I watched the birds and the weather moving across the sky, the shadows of the clouds, the birds, moving across the water. I almost felt that I was out there, as much on the sea as on my bed, that I could see the movement of the fish beneath the waters.

And maybe it sounds a little crazy, maybe it was. The edges between reality and unreality seemed blurred since the Haemorrhage... the sides of roads dissolving and moving in my peripheral vision, nothing quite as it seemed. Walls closing in on me, sometimes with loud music, I seemed to be able to see the sound. And my brain was still able to reflect and see, and to understand what I was seeing and doing. But I was aware of how easily the thread between a rational and factual way of thinking and a more dreamlike feeling world could be cut. And a part of me, the thinking part, knew that I had to keep that thread intact, to keep the thinking part of me strong, not to succumb to the lure of just letting go and sensing. That way I would not 'recover', I would need more and more caring for. This was one of those moments of choice.

'I took the one less travelled by – and that has made all the difference' (Robert Frost, *The Road Not Taken*).

And I thought that my task now was to identify what went on for me and I wrote a list of how I thought I was helping my thinking brain to grow:

- In the constant reflecting and recording in my Journals.
- The reading and learning of poems by memory.
- Doing Jigsaws, choosing and placing the pieces to make the whole picture.
- The Game of Patience, focussing attention over and over.
- Stitching the Wedding Tapestry, choosing colours, designing, thinking.

Later I relearn how to crochet and make a large blanket, each stitch a meditation.

And I thought of that great desire I had to play Games, often so tiresome for my patient family whose first choice of activity is definitely not to play Snap or Woodland Happy Families or throw dice for Yams or Ludo! And of course I see now why that was, indeed is, so attractive to me. Emotionally there is the enjoyment of returning to a favourite childhood pastime – but that would usually quickly be filled. Now it had an added gain for me. Taking turns, making easy decisions, noticing, remembering… there are the skills involved and of course these games are designed and popular because they help children's brains to grow. And also there was the nurturing and enjoyment of engaging in an activity with others, the laughter, the pleasure. Because perhaps there were so many things that I couldn't do – would have done before with family and friends. Long walks. Evenings in noisy restaurants or somewhere that had music playing. Going to a friend's party. Visits out. Driving or taking a train or flying to meetings, for holidays. I was too slow, too tired, too easily overwhelmed to travel or to take part.

So these seemingly unimportant small things had two functions – to build my brain, the concentration, recognition, bringing attention, whether to a card, a die, a move on a board. All need thinking and reasoning as well as intuition. And at this time, when I found it difficult to converse and I felt rather useless and cut off, it was a good way to be with others in a structured way. (Maybe that was part of why I chatted away to a stranger on the bus!)

I was used to being a certain way and my family and friends and work colleagues were used to me being a certain way and all of us were trying to make our way through the cloying mud of the Tsunami, the markers all gone. Because I had changed. So a game for me gave companionship, some rules within which to communicate, play the game of communication, as well as the channels in which to think.

I found it so terribly hard, and often heart wrenching, to be with people I loved and had lived or worked with. It was with them at this time that I was most aware of how different I was.

I wanted to be back as I had been.

They wanted me to be back as I had been.

And we were learning to meet where we were now… all of us. It is not an easy journey for anyone.

I wanted to reach out and try to grasp them, but I probably didn't as at the same time as I was trying to build MY coping self, the desperate urge not to be dependent. To push push push to Recover – to keep my Thinking. I could see how easily it could all just dissolve and fall away from me.

I could feel the determination in me and I understood it through my body, poems and drawings. And I began to draw my journey.

I fought. I built my brain. I learned poems and listened to Podcasts of Talks and I read stories. I relearnt how to go online and to send emails, eventually to order food online and have it delivered. And experienced again human kindness – how incredibly kind Tesco's Delivery Men were when I was at my most confused and exhausted. One day they brought it all into my kitchen and he took one look at me and said 'why don't you sit down and tell us where to put it', and they put it all away in the cupboards. And I met with so many acts of kindness like that, often when not expected.

And I went out and walked with my stick, explored further and decided that I wanted to get another dog to be a companion and to accompany me on my walks, to run in the woods and on the beaches. My very dear border collie Timmy had died last year and I missed him. I missed the structure too of having to go out for a walk, having another creature to look after and care for.

I was ready for the next phase of my journey, I was in the foothills of the mountains and over the empty plain. I began to drive – very difficult – it was like being a learner driver all over again.

This was a massive step – it could well have been too terrifying but I was able to step back into some of that Automatic pilot without which many of the things we do would simply to be too exhausting.

Chapter 7: The Way Lies over the Mountains

Driving is very different from all my other re-learnt activities in that it is potentially dangerous. I had that very new learner fear, but I was lucky – I had a dear friend, Janet, who was for many years a driving instructor, and she came out with me.

It felt very jerky at first, rather like so many years ago when I first got in a car to drive. But actually, when I stopped being scared and thinking about it, auto-pilot did kick in and my body knew how to release the clutch – I automatically felt my way through changing the gears in response to the sense of what the car needed. I could still do this, just as I could still eat, put food in my mouth, clean my teeth and so on. Clumsier, slower, but all still there.

That was a huge relief and I even found when we went out into busier roads that again I could automatically judge distance – be aware of other traffic – when to signal – when to pull out.

So far so good. The far more difficult thing was, as ever, unexpected. I didn't have much sense of speed… so kept realising I was only doing 30 or 40 mph and needed to go faster. And judging an appropriate speed continued to need constant attention.

I needed to know where I was going and ideally be on a familiar route – I could not easily make sudden route change decisions while driving. I also seemed to have lost the ability to follow a map.

I found busy roundabouts challenging. You have to be aware of so much and I found it hard to be aware of what was coming from my right or left at the same time. So I was slow, and that eventually led me to only driving at quiet times of day and on familiar routes and not much above 50mph – and never at night because the glare of lights took my attention and was exhausting.

So I learned in a new way that the level of multi-tasking involved in driving is immense and I needed to account for that, drive short distances and rest.

Later, I discovered that if a diversion or something else that needed a change in direction occurred, I could not manage that and would have to stop as soon as I could. I realised that I needed my attention to be at a high level and that our auto-pilot is what helps us to drive easily. Mine was reduced so I felt I was constantly driving as a new driver. It amazed me to realise that we all do this all the time, and how much we automatically push the boundaries of our attention in everyday life.

So I drove less; if I needed to go farther or in the dark I would get a train or bus – I became an expert on non-car travelling!

This all affected my life in a number of ways… before the Haemorrhage I had travelled a lot, often abroad, up and down the country… to Scotland, to Cornwall – to work, to deliver training courses in psychotherapy and mindfulness or to visit friends.

But that had all gone, I could visit by train, but it is very different… the spontaneity and control I had had was gone. And I could not travel abroad – I would need a 'minder', I knew, just to negotiate airports.

Having a Brain Injury, I was discovering, brings us up against the reality of how many skills we just take for granted to live our everyday lives. It was a loss I felt keenly – that ability to just choose to nip here or there – go on an unexpected journey or visit. I didn't NIP anywhere now – everything needed, and still needs to some extent, to be planned.

I was referred for Cognitive Testing to see if and when I would be ready to go back to work. I had weddings to plan for. I would look for a puppy. I knew what sort of dog I wanted – I wanted a Whippet.

Chapter 8: Living in the View From My Window

'What is essential is invisible to the eye'
(Antoine de Saint-Exupéry, *The Little Prince*)

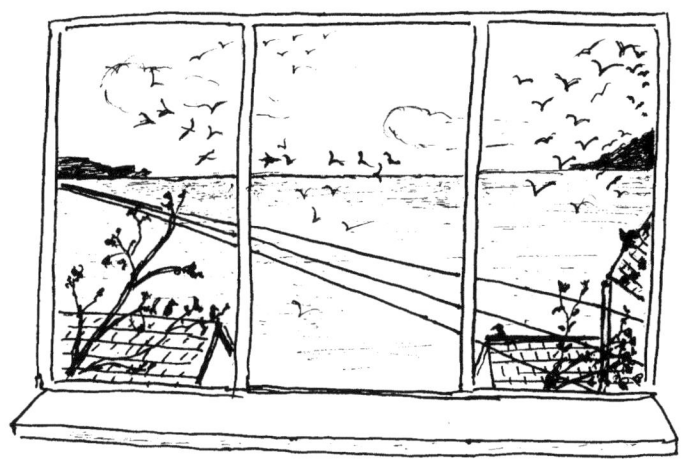

As I become accustomed to being home, I begin to feel as if I have found my centre – a gradual dropping into me – my body. Is this how it is? Is this how I am going to be now? I feel a curiosity about who and what I am now. Realising that alongside the physical aches and pains – the occasional periods of agitation – there is an awareness of this moment and ME – as I am now. Sitting in this bed that is so familiar and yet now I see everything with New Eyes – it is familiar and yet all totally new. The view through my window – of the roofs – the trees – the sea and islands and the sky – How come I didn't notice before how it all changes every moment – had I ever noticed before how beautiful the terracotta chimney pots are – silhouetted against the blue of the sea? The different leaves and shapes of the leaves – how the trees move with the clouds in the sky – a dance of life – birds alighting – pausing – flying. Watching one windy morning how a jackdaw seems to almost be flying backwards as it struggled in a high wind.

I felt as though I could happily spend the rest of my life just contemplating this view – how come I had never noticed it in all its wonderful detail before – this view that I have looked at every day for at least the last 10 years.

And I bring my attention back to the weight of my body connected and supported by my bed – appreciating too, perhaps fully for the first time, the beauty of the height of it and the turquoise curled Victorian bed ends – this was an old Victorian bedstead – also however very high – so not so easy for getting on – or, as I was now, falling or climbing on and off with difficulty!

And as I come back into the body – from my journey through the window, I also am aware again of the constant exhaustion and pain. That to do anything, to get up now, go downstairs – involved me really thinking about how to do it – not quite like the first time – I could ride the bike of walking and moving now – but my balance and sense of direction and speed was none too good!

This may seem a lot about nothing very much – so I would have thought once – 'get on with it – the story – what happened next?'

But the gift of my experience – and the Mindfulness practice that stayed there for me in my body – was supporting me in just being with these moments – not trying to ignore or push them away or to 'be better'. There were things that helped me to be more comfortable – certainly pain killers – but also my practice – and the new gift of noticing the wonder of each moment – each new sight. I was not so caught up in jumbles of thought – planning this and that – remembering this and that – worrying about this and that – regretting… wishing… hoping… There was really just this moment – and curiosity about that – and from somewhere a trust that somehow I could learn to be with this.

Slowly I began to do more – the name is always on everyone's tongue. Recovery. It has always puzzled me – and still does – what is it that I am recovering? Did I lose something? Is it just behind a veil – invisible – or gone – where? And who am I – this question of who am I – where am I – just now and then something will happen and I will remember and wonder – there is always the mirror – looking into my eyes sometimes, as I did back then at the beginning in the Hospital bathroom mirror. Where are you – looking deep into my eyes. Where are you? Are you in there? Pink Floyd song – is there anybody in there? Yes – the ME that I am in this moment – not confined by an identity or an expectation. I am just my experience – and that seems enough.

Quite frequently my brain would 'slip' – I could feel it as a sensation, sometimes a slipping in my head – or a sense as if a chunk of something just broke away and fell away somewhere. I knew it could have been frightening – but I was too exhausted with bothering to think about it very much – and just noticing was fine – that's how it is, that's how I am right now.

I imagine my mindfulness practice had something to do with this acceptance – other people over the years have been far more concerned by apparent changes in me than I ever have.

It was as though there was a dance of the increased awareness of sensation – spaciousness and loss of time that had come with the haemorrhage, and the awareness of sensation and spaciousness that comes with meditation practices.

However, there were times when I became distressed by the inability I had to focus on anything for very long. But looking back right there in intensive care at the very beginning – like the beginning of birth – I was able to be aware of the breath moving in my body – and feel a sense of compassion in its presence. And now I wonder if the years of meditation practice did make a difference… and that although it was weeks before I could deliberately lead myself through a familiar practice – either a Body Scan – moving attention around the body – or a Sitting practice – watching each movement of the breath and the coming and going of thoughts – I was aware of the weight of the body and contact with the bed or feet with the floor – and the fact that I was breathing.

I began to wonder about how other people who have Brain Haemorrhages or some other form of, particularly, Brain Injury might access this – could they learn to do this? Without this ability to notice without judgement, to be able to ground myself in moments of confusion and pain, to know how to move my attention from pain to the contact of the body with bed and not get so caught up in the pain – allowing it to be there but not engaging in pushing and wanting it to go… which of course generally just makes it stay longer and be felt more deeply.

So my mindfulness practice was very much a part of my experience right from the beginning – the Tsunami of the Brain on the stairs of my house – the potentially frightening and certainly unpleasant hospital procedures – the discovery that I was changed – the pain and struggles and losses that were to come… made so much more bearable through the physical grounding of the practices and the attitudes that come with it – compassion – acceptance – curiosity.

Neuro Notes 2: Making Progress

Recovery tends to slow down after a few months, and later stages are sometimes more difficult.

The person's awareness of their difficulties may increase as they feel better and try to do more. Although this growing awareness is part of recovery, it can often cause distress and sadness. People may feel discouraged and despondent.

Difficulties caused by changes in the brain are beyond the person's control. Nevertheless, they may feel they are 'stupid' or 'useless' or even 'crazy', and blame themselves when it is clearly not their fault.

Optimism and hope for a full recovery may fade. People rarely recover completely and return to exactly the way they were before.

This realisation can trigger a grief reaction, anger, or low mood. Many people become depressed after a stroke or a traumatic brain injury.

Anxiety is also very common, and can be a barrier to recovery and rehabilitation. Avoiding things because of anxiety creates more anxiety and more avoidance. People need understanding and support to help them to do as much as possible despite feeling anxious.

Natural recovery slows down after about six months, and again after two years. However, improvements can continue for much longer. Other parts of the brain can take over from injured areas, and brain tissue can sometimes repair itself.

Learning to get around the difficulties is also part of recovery. People who keep trying to improve, and to work around their difficulties, and who have supportive family or friends, tend to do well in the long-term.

Having a goal to aim for can be very helpful. Goals should be realistic and based on things that improve with practice. Making progress will boost the person's confidence and encourage them.

Practicing long-standing skills and abilities can also be helpful and positive. Some things may come back surprisingly easily – the 'muscle memory' may still be strong. Old skills may be linked to happy memories, and bring out feelings of confidence and capability.

Part 3: Over the Mountains

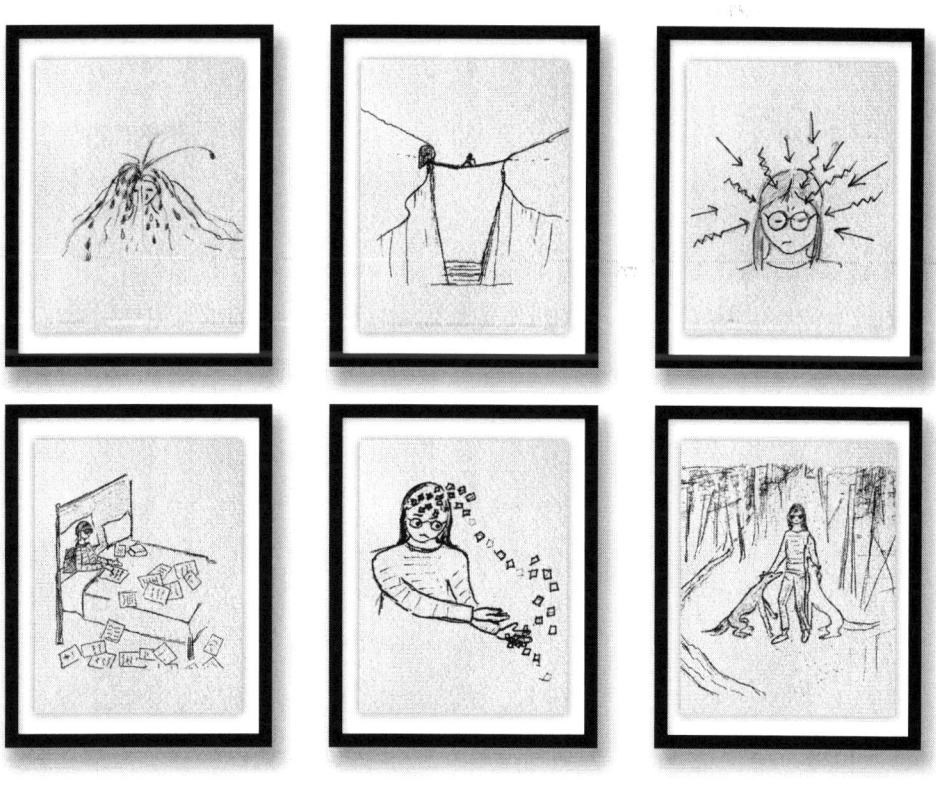

Chapter 9: The Cup

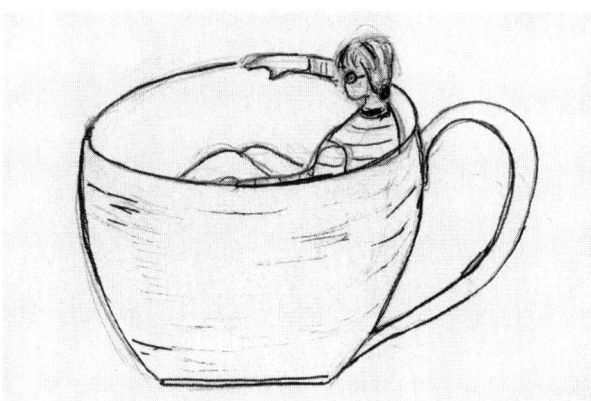

There are many challenges that have come with the changes from the Haemorrhage. In my Cognitive testing I begin to understand it in terms of the Brain Injury I have received – and how I am finding my way around this new brain – just like the mud choked roads and houses in the Tsunami.

And there were so many difficult and challenging situations – that perception of the loudness and speed of the environment I found myself in – and also just turning towards curiosity about my experience, not pushing it away – and noticing that, as well as the dark over-bright and loud difficult times, there were the quiet times of beauty. Those times when I was overtaken by the environment – the lights, the movement of the roads… new decisions… not recognising familiar faces – my world had changed.

My support came from that view from my window – watching the changing of the weather – the seasons.

Sitting up in my bed – a refuge to return to – the beauty of the birds flying past – the sea… changing… the sky… changing… the trees… gently moving in the breeze.

And the joy of Poetry that seemed to just capture all the changes and difficulties that emerged.

'All things pass – the sunrise does not last all morning… the cloudburst does not last all day.'
(Lao Tzu)

Chapter 9: The Cup

And my Mindfulness practices – somewhere I could always turn to if things became too much.

Every day is a fresh beginning
Listen, my soul, to the glad refrain
And, spite of old sorrow and older sinning
And puzzles forecasted and possible pain
Take heart with the day, and begin again.
(Susan Coolidge) from the last verse of *New Every Morning*

But as I went out more – learned to drive farther – to shop for food – to begin to think about going back to work – learning to expect the flashing lights, moving objects around me... I yearned for calm and peace – and one day I saw this picture of a Cup that I had painted some years ago... I have it still and it was given to me by one of my Mindfulness Training Groups at the end of a course – it is beautiful – white ceramic with swirly design – cool to hold – and seems spacious. I imagined myself being able to climb into such a space and just sit there – supported by the curved sides of the cup – all the loud sounds and flashing objects seen out of the corner of my eyes would be calmed – somewhere to rest for a while within the chaos of my head.

I took the cup with me in my imagination everywhere – and whenever I was lost or confused or overwhelmed I would imagine I was resting in the cup... protected. I needed something concrete – not just an idea of being held but an image.

And this became really helpful in the difficult situations, being with people who don't understand or who expect me to be as I've always been. And the sadness and loss and distress I would feel. I would remember my cup, feeling its smoothness as if I was in the cup, held and contained. And I was able to return to that sense of connection I'd had when first going out after hospital. My refuge in just holding my cup.

And now another gain from the Haemorrhage and the changes to my brain seemed to be how connected I found I was with other people – anyone I talked to – that deep sense of knowing them... it was as if the barriers that come from conventions were not there and wherever I was – whether I had met them before or not – there were people – open, kind, friendly. The sense of connection that I felt with people was so strong.

There was a sense of Acceptance here now – I was no longer fighting against my experience but simply accepting that this is the way things are...

I felt surrounded by love – even the occasional shock of others not understanding – I seemed able to respond to their difficulties with compassion... I could see that it was not easy for people – they wanted me to be the same – they tried to understand me in terms of their experience (as we all do) but they could not generally see how I saw – I had new eyes – I was in a new and different world – like a parallel universe, and we conversed between the two.

And as time went by I could read more – I had always been a keen reader and I found with joy that I could still follow a story – and the first book I read – which I had read before – was Laurie Lee's *When I Walked out One Midsummer Morning*, and his writing is very poetic – I found that I could either read fact-based books or novels that were lyrical.

Life seemed leisurely – in fact I had little sense of time – no hurry and no delay – and I began to actively search for a puppy – and that led to me driving one day out to a smallholding to look at some Whippet puppies – and then, a few weeks later, to bring home Toby – nine weeks old – the warmth and joy of a new puppy. He would become my companion from now on – someone other than me to care for – to put first.

So by the time I decided to try a day a week back at work I began to know the territory of Sub Arachnoid recovery. Some of the difficulties in perception, energy and memory had all surfaced – and I had found some support strategies – my practice – the cup – my Toby.

There were times when back at work that I felt so strongly the loss of who I was – what I was – the knowledge I had – and at times I would grieve for that lost me. And I struggle as I begin to find out all the ways in which I have changed... the exhaustion of trying to compensate and to build a new professional me.

And so much is coming up in family too now – K and F are going to have a baby – a new baby for the family and they too are going to get married – so two weddings to plan for now. So exciting.

Plans are now in full swing for D and C's wedding. After a month or so in work I go down to Brighton again – similar difficulties in travelling – the overwhelm of people – train timetable boards flashing – the noise of announcements – making choices... the overload of the lights and noise of voices in carriages – wanting to curl up in a ball on the floor of the train – but instead closing my eyes, imagining myself held in my cup – breathing in... breathing out – just this moment... just this moment.

And in Brighton – a shock again – I think I had imagined it would all be back to normal on this visit... but now – although I could find my way around better – I still could only endure being in places without too much noise and where I felt the environment to be spacious – I still tired so easily – and found it so hard to participate in any conversation with more than one person – overwhelming – exhausting. And also more able to recognise where I was going – to achieve and buy what I needed.

Often I felt content – connected – enjoying the benefits – the increased pleasure in my new activities – poems… walking my puppy… reading… sewing… being with my team of dear friends and colleagues in the University – the Mindfulness Centre, but also the awful ruptures – not being understood – not understanding – getting lost – getting so exhausted that I seemed to simply shut down.

Quite early on, it was time for our Mindfulness Centre Conference – this was something I had initiated and set up before the Haemorrhage last year, and my team had taken forward. It was wonderful and strange to go to it – this changed me – walking now on a stick – to me my face was so different. And it was an interesting time because, looking back, I can see that I was able to do the things that were my strengths, but that there were areas where I was quite unable to participate. I could introduce the Conference – stand up and talk – and talk to people individually. But I couldn't find my way around – I needed someone with me to both tell me where and when I was meant to be somewhere and to show me how to get there.

And the crash came – and it was a terrible shock this first time; afterwards, I was to anticipate and get used to it – going into a crowded room of chairs to listen to a presentation – finding I was unable to follow anything much – there was too much going on – too many people – I could not bear the brightness of the screens showing diagrams and writing – everything started to move around – I was sick and dizzy and had to ask my colleague to help me to get out. Once in a room, I tended not to be able to easily find how to get out. The walls would close in – the noise grow louder – the lights unbearably bright and in the corner of my vision, movement… arrows darting… a buzzing noise in my head.

I crashed – or what I came to think of as crashing – and it took several days for me to recover.

It was a shock and I became more cautious about going out… and even more about going IN – the insides of buildings were even more unpredictable than outside – at least outside there was space; inside the space closed in.
I used my image of the cup – to imagine that I was held within the cup so if I began to feel the shifting around me, I imagined the feeling of sitting in the cup, supported, quiet; no sound or moving lights could get in there.

Chapter 10: Back to Work and Cognitive Testing

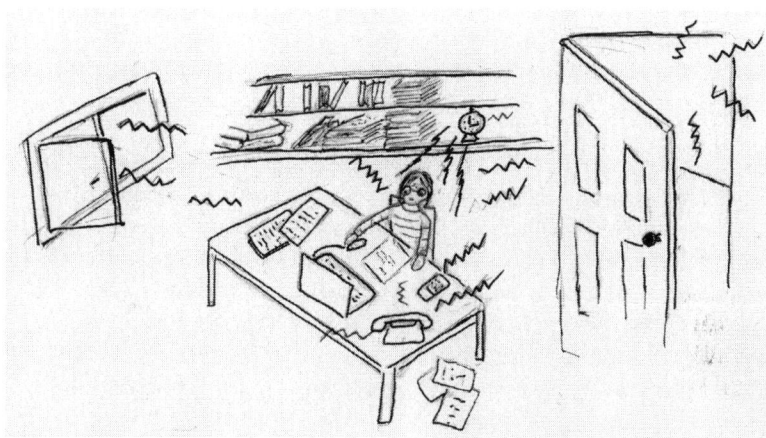

Things seem to be moving fast now. I am managing most everyday tasks better. A lot of my attention has gone into building my brain up – I am learning poems – every day a new poem, such pleasure in the learning and reciting of them – that sense of almost 'eating' them, they are inside me. My brain is Hungry to learn.

I am also trying to relearn some of the early scales and tunes I used to play on the piano – but that is very halting; my fingers don't seem to respond as I want them to. Because of that it is overtiring so I decide to concentrate on what seems helpful.

The planned Cognitive Testing will give us a sense of whether I can manage the return to work now – and I am quite scared that maybe as I add more to my brain I may lose my poems – I hope not – they are so helpful to me. To just carry around a book of poems in my head! Or lose the person I am now – go into a sort of no person land.

I now really needed to be driving again and so my driving instructor friend Janet helped me to adjust back into driving and gave me feedback where needed. Now I drove the 11 miles on my own to Colwyn Bay for Cognitive Testing at the Brain Injury Clinic. At first I was very aware of movement in my peripheral vision – I had to learn how to shut that out… But by the end of the drive it was already less intrusive. Actually, we see everything we move past out of the corner of both eyes as we drive – but we filter it and only look and focus where we need to. But I couldn't do that and so everything could be over tiring. And already some of that auto-pilot was kicking in but I quickly found that I could not widen my attention beyond the task of driving and that I could not put my attention on driving and listening to the radio or music. So I just drove.

Because I knew from the past where I was going I was actually able to arrive there – following directions would probably have been too much – constant divided attention.

As usual, just going into a new building was challenging. I am so impacted by whatever building I am in – this building had a lot of corridors – doors to go through – a waiting area with comings and goings. I manage this immediate impression of where I am by deliberately bringing my mindfulness practice to whatever is going on for me. So, walking through the door – anxiety at not knowing where to go – sitting in the waiting area with things moving at the edge of my vision, sometimes as if the wall was leaning in a bit, confusion at every door as I go down the corridor – does it open this way or that? And then the view on the other side of the door – is this corridor going to close on me? Then into a room with a large table that seems to feel all the space. Sitting down with H, my neuropsychologist at what was to be the beginning – although I did not know it then – of a long journey together. Looking back I can see that without her, my recovery could have been very different… her quiet understanding and reflection began to help me for the first time to understand and put into context what had happened to me. To begin to learn and understand what it means to have a Brain Injury and learn how I could respond to the many difficulties that came up for me.

The Cognitive Testing was exhausting – but I was working with this very skilled and supportive lady… I felt very fortunate. Extraordinary patience as I repeated myself, forgot, stumbled over and over and probably talked far too much – I know I repeat and that this is a feature of this sort of brain injury.

And then the next week I travel again, alone on the train to Liverpool for an MRI Scan. I know the route now – can hold it in my head but travelling it still requires me to be aware of each step – each change of train – the route up and down escalators – massive – so massive what we usually do it without thinking – and that is just the getting there. I have to bring my attention and a strong effort into every step to the long escalators, to stepping onto the escalator, to filtering out everything going on around me… all the people – or, even worse, empty corridors with no indications of where I am going. Then the finding of the right platform, decisions to get on and off trains. Will I ever get used to this again? It is an exhausting process. If one thing happens to interrupt it, then I lose attention and... the only word for it really... is Crash. And there are different levels of The Crash, I discover. Now I become aware of it when I realise I cannot think, my brain seems to have stopped – I am not too sure where I am or where I am going. The only thing to do is to find somewhere to sit down and do a Mindfulness practice to settle and let go. And gradually I will settle and the thinking starts again – a bit slow – but I will recognise where I am and can take the next steps. If there is time and anywhere to go for a cup of tea or coffee, then that is even better.

I learn from working with H that this is normal – the territory of brain injury. I need to learn to accept this as just how it is – much of the distress certainly comes from fear and wanting things to be different and not understanding why I am having these experiences. My mindfulness practice needs to invite more Acceptance, I REALISE – This IS how it is. It is no good wanting or waiting for anything to change... it probably will, but I am not going to return to how and who I was before. This is How and Who I am – being curious – opening to how it is NOW – letting go of HOW IT WAS THEN.

Now that I know more about the territory of brain injury, I realise that the conditions I went back into at work were not helpful. In my absence the whole department had moved into a new office... and so my old room had gone, all my files had been moved, all the notices on the board gone. Nothing was as I remembered it.

I had been on my own and now I was sharing an office – and everything had been moved. This is what you would expect with a move of office when you are not there – and picking up the pieces would always have difficulties – but one of the effects of my brain injury I was finding increasingly was that I needed things to stay the same, I could not manage anything being moved to a new place – my brain simply seemed unable to hold the change. I found that very distressing. As though all my anchor points, my reference points to remember where things were, what was currently active, all were in confusion.

I found too that I was no longer able to manage the filing system – once something was out of sight it did not exist. I no longer put things in drawers – it all had to be on my desk – labelled – in sight. Just that was enough to make my return very difficult for me, and for others too.

Sharing a room too was difficult – I was easily distracted – I could not do one task while someone else was on the phone or even typing.

With help from my wonderful colleagues and Office Manager I began to be updated on where we were – to pick up some of the threads of my work, to see the whole picture. There were many challenges. But not what I might have expected – picking up where I had left off was not going to be easy –

and perhaps not possible – I saw with new eyes, thought with a new brain – remembered in new ways, and I had to find out what they were.

After a few weeks I moved into an office on my own and began to organise everything in piles that I could see. I had to be very structured.

I found bright overhead lights hurtful to my eyes so my office was most comfortable with the blinds down and very low lighting – not so good for others coming to a meeting perhaps! Gradually I was arriving back.

I found talking to people, being in and even chairing a meeting quite easy – communicating, relating to others was not so different – although I needed a lot of prompting around what we were going to talk about and I needed to be clear on exactly what the subject was and not have any changes. So I was also finding out the way my new brain worked. I also began slowly to find out that once a decision had been made I would not necessarily remember it – or what we had talked about – and so again I had to find other memory prompts which I had not needed before.

One thing that was very difficult for me was how many tasks I could manage at one time. Once (I thought) I had been excellent at multi-tasking. Not anymore. I came to describe this process as a bowl of Oranges. It was as if I had a bowl on my Desk with oranges in. I could just about manage two oranges – two different topics or things on a list. But somehow if there were three or more, it became unmanageable.

I would sit down at my desk with Task A and B to do. I would work on A and know that B was next. But if someone came in and either asked me to do something else, or just put down some papers or a message on my desk – a third orange – then I could feel it all falling in my head, as if there were too many oranges for the bowl and they all just tumbled to the floor and I couldn't remember any of them.

It took me a little while to realise what was happening, and then the Orange Bowl metaphor helped me to recognise it as it happened. It was a useful metaphor because of course I recognised that this happened at home too – with lists of what to buy – what to do. So I started trying to get everyone to recognise this – to not come in and give me one more thing. But the workplace is made up of 'things waiting to be done' or overflowing bowls of oranges. And as this went on, not only the oranges and my memory of what I was doing would go, but, as the daily work of managing a team and University Research Department began to unfold, so my brain struggled. The sense of crashing became familiar. I began to recognise it – and, as ever, my Mindfulness Practice helped.

The first signs were a sense of slipping... familiar now... in my head, my face would feel somehow different, jaw slack, breath slow, I would have a sense almost of falling sometimes. My Practice helped me to recognise when this started to happen, and then I would do a Settling Practice.

SETTLING PRACTICE
Notice myself sitting or standing wherever I am
Notice and allow the sensations in the head and the body
Lengthen my posture and feel my feet on the floor and body on the chair
(if sitting)
And then bringing my attention to my breath
Following each in breath and each out breath
This breath all the way in – relaxing.
This breath all the way out – letting go.
Doing this for a few minutes.

I found this would help me to let go of the tensions, for my brain to clear a little so I could carry on.

Chapter 11: Living in my Brain

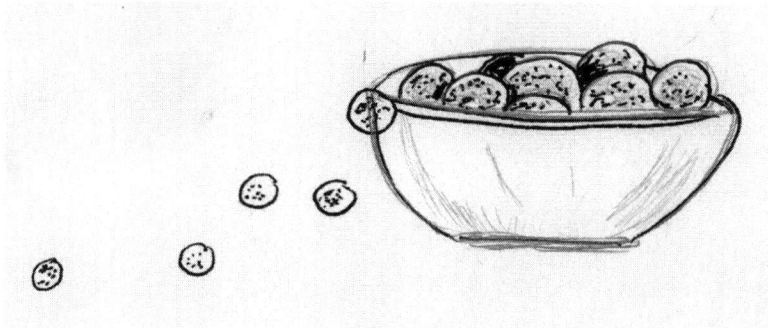

I have new coping techniques. It is a late Easter this year, the end of April, and my new puppy Toby is with me – structuring my day for me – a companion – he demands attention and activity but does not require me to think!

I am tired. I always seem to be so tired. And I decide that I need Plans – Strategies for managing my Brain.

I remember the Jackdaw that I saw – managing to fly on a stormy blustery day – his feathers blown forwards as he seemed to be pulled backwards by the wind but somehow struggling on, letting the strong gust of wind take him and then flying backwards when he needed to and gradually moving forwards until the gust subsided. He rode the wind, however it blew. And I needed to do that. How was I going to learn to rest my brain – to find a way to ride the winds of constant information and demands made on the brain… to rest between the blasts of thought?

And I have a growing bunch of strategies now. And most of them are VISUAL – so the pictures are then more likely to remain in my Brain. I am more likely to remember if an image is attached to something.

I think of the day as moving constantly between clock times – times I need to be DOING – and times I need to sustain myself by BEING… Cup time. To build in these times to pause and rest. Otherwise I will crash.

Another way I think about using oranges was to think of them as tasks. How many oranges can I hold in my hands at once? How many do I choose to accept or pick up? I can manage one – sometimes two. But with two they can be confused; any more and they will tumble away out of my mind. A reminder for me to just do one thing at a time.

And so I move on – I am writing… teaching… developing our Mindfulness Supervision Model… and as long as I keep these tasks separate and only do each for a short time with rests between, I am beginning to manage – to DO. I feel I am back… I am changed, but I hope that by developing these strategies in response to how my brain reacts now and with my mindfulness practice helping me to notice, I can pause and rest frequently – and notice when the fears and dark thoughts arise, to have a way to let go… Without that I think I would have been overwhelmed.

So my day plan is:
Rest
Only do one thing at a time
Only put one thing on the waiting list
Noticing when I begin to tire
Stopping and taking Cup time out
Pausing every so often for a drink and to sit and breathe.

And it was important for my colleagues to support my way of working because if I did not manage distraction, everything was likely to just fall away and I would not know what I was doing or had done.

And perhaps the most useful part of my Mindfulness practice has been Noticing, noticing thoughts and doubts, not grabbing them or pushing them away as we so often do. I would just fall down a funnel then, caught in thoughts, doubts, fears, wants.

And once again my bedroom view brought me wisdom.

One morning as I looked out over the sea before going to work I noticed how windy it was out there.

A large grey cloud was moving quite quickly across the early morning sky. First one dark cloud and then another, each one getting darker and darker and moving swiftly… Followed by others, less distinct… filling the sky. And they were like my thoughts for the day – I had a lot to do, was worried, will I manage?… and my thoughts were just like these clouds – moving over the sky and away. I did not have to go with them. I could just notice them and let them go, and let my worries and fears go too.

All things pass. Even this. Just let go.

And that became a strong practice for me and I learned, and others around me learned, a new post-brain injury way of working.

Life is always bringing us difficulties and challenges, as Jon Kabat-Zinn writes about in 'Full Catastrophe Living'.

And as I learn to accept, this changed me. I realise too that I need a certain attitude, one of accepting myself as I am, rather than trying to change to be the person I was, or that other people want. And I make a list of some of the things that can happen daily and that I want to respond to by noticing and accepting.

NOTICING AND ACCEPTING
To welcome whatever comes:
Each new puppy puddle on the floor
Each new complexity
Each new work dilemma
Each new email
Each time I realise I have forgotten something or done something wrong
To remember that to be alive is to open the door to challenges and difficulties every day, whatever they are.

Chapter 12: When Getting Better is Getting Worse

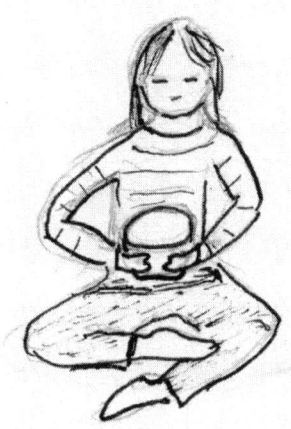

I feel in a lost middle place – neither completely ill nor completely well. People seem to peer at me, enquiringly, as though they are looking for something – or somebody. What do they see? It is hard to be in this middle place.

I often turn to my Mindfulness practice; the breathing calms and settles me. And when the pain in my head nags away and sometimes grows intense, I breathe into that too – and it makes it manageable – present still, but not so intense, it seems to soften.

Some months ago, I could only be 'in the present' – things are changing now. As I 'get better' I can do more… I am coming back into my life – and in a way that highlights the changes and I am 'getting worse'.

Despite all the pain and confusion I was in, there has also been that sense of 'new eyes'… I have been so involved in just being in the world I see… the sky… clouds, birds and wind and rain. Everything so present. Noticing the detail and beauty of even the tiles on the roof opposite – and the wonder of the birds – as they balanced on the wind. And as I came back into being more active in this material world, the wind – that perception of the intensity of colour – sights – that early vivid perception, began to fade. And I felt the loss.

And as weeks went on, I realised that all the intensity of that early perception would fade, the brightness of the 'in between place' that existed near to the haemorrhage would fade. A mist descends over the memory – yet when the mist parts or lifts, it is still there – squeezing through the cracks of everyday life.

And as I go back into the Work World – I can take this with me.

I have been changed. My brain works differently in many ways – slower – finding previously easy tasks difficult – and also I can see a new path through… the New Eyes are still with me.

And I am beginning to realise more and more that other people (and I am sure I would have been the same) have not changed and they are looking for the old me to come back. They respond to me as I was – and then I think it can be hard to see the changes, or see them as positives, perhaps.

And I find, as I have to relate more and more with other people – groups of people, after my relatively secluded recovery… that I am different.

I cannot respond in the same way to people. For instance, in asking me a lot of questions about something… which previously I would have answered immediately – moving effortlessly from one subject to another… now I could not do that.

I need to go slowly. And to answer or deal with just one question or issue at a time… and then I need space between subjects or they just blend into one. I can only hold one question at a time or they will all tumble away – I cannot link them and I do not remember what I have just answered – unless there is space.

I feel people's exasperation – and often they come with plans for how I can deal with this – and these are hard to grasp too. For the Mindfulness Centre to go at my pace, we would all have to slow down quite a bit. That is not going to happen – and I find myself putting huge pressure on me to speed up. I should concentrate more. Try harder.

And of course that just results in further crashing and exhaustion. And I realise this was to be expected. And maybe I expected everyone to understand just how it was for me. But how can they? I begin to doubt myself – can I do this? – and, more importantly, should I be doing this?

I go home that night and the Tesco delivery man arrives and unloads all the food for me to put away – and I 'crash' completely. That awful feeling of everything going, falling away from me and that strange feeling in my head that has become familiar of great slabs of brain slipping, slipping away.

And this passes. I am beginning to learn that this happens when I do too much – this was about a day at work and then coming home to home tasks… as I have done most days for years. But something had changed, I had to find ways to steer myself through.

I was learning how to be in the world with a brain injury.

And also how to be in the world, at work with other people. I see doubt in their eyes – I often give them too much information about what is going on… although I do not want to hide or pretend… but there is something it seems that is unsettling in a person changing AS a person – it is unseen, unpredictable, unlooked for. Sometimes I see the alarm in their eyes, or a shutter coming down. And partly this interests me, that observing part that seems so strong now in this new me… What is happening? How it is happening? How can I respond… for me and for them?

And as I go back regularly now to work, my SPACE recedes… my CUP fills up with tasks and thoughts – choices.

I began to do a daily CUP Reflection Practice.

CUP PRACTICE
I take my spacious cup or bowl and sit on a chair, or bed, or any where I am supported.
And I bring my attention to my body sitting here.
Feel the contact of the body on the seat / bed / chair.
And Feel the contact of my hands holding the Cup.
And I bring attention to my breath.
Following and noticing the in breath and out breath.
Allowing this to be a space to rest and just let be –
As if held and cradled by the cup.
Allowing the ups and downs and difficulties that may be here.

Neuro Notes 3: Coping with Memory and Concentration Problems

A stroke or brain injury is likely to affect concentration, memory, and the ability to organise things. It can be helpful to:

Do one thing at a time.

Do anything difficult in a quiet place, where there will be no distractions or interruptions.

Do things when you are feeling alert and have the most energy. Take breaks when you need to. Start early so that you are not under time pressure.

Plan the day or week ahead using a diary, calendar or whiteboard. Decisions can be easier with a list of the advantages and disadvantages of each choice.

Difficult tasks are less overwhelming when broken down into stages or steps. It can help to write each one down, and to think about one at a time.

Coping with fatigue and difficult emotions

A stroke or brain injury can also affect emotions, behaviour and personality. The changes may be severe and unchanging, or they may improve slowly.

Emotions may come to the surface quickly. The person may be easily upset, angry or frustrated. These changes are less obvious than physical limitations, but are often more difficult to cope with. Stopping to take some slow deep breaths when things are difficult can be a good coping strategy.

A stroke or brain injury also causes fatigue and exhaustion which can make emotional responses more intense and more difficult. Taking time out in midst of these challenges – such as a mindful breathing space – can be a lifeline.

Stopping to rest, and taking time out can help to restore energy and enthusiasm, lift mood, and prevent a crisis, such as a panic attack or an emotional 'meltdown'. A short mindfulness practice whilst sitting quietly can be an effective way of managing a difficult or overwhelming situation, reducing anxiety, or making pain more tolerable.

Jody felt safe and more contained when she imagined herself sitting inside her spacious cup. Imagining beautiful or calm surroundings can have the same effect.

Part 4: Down into a New World

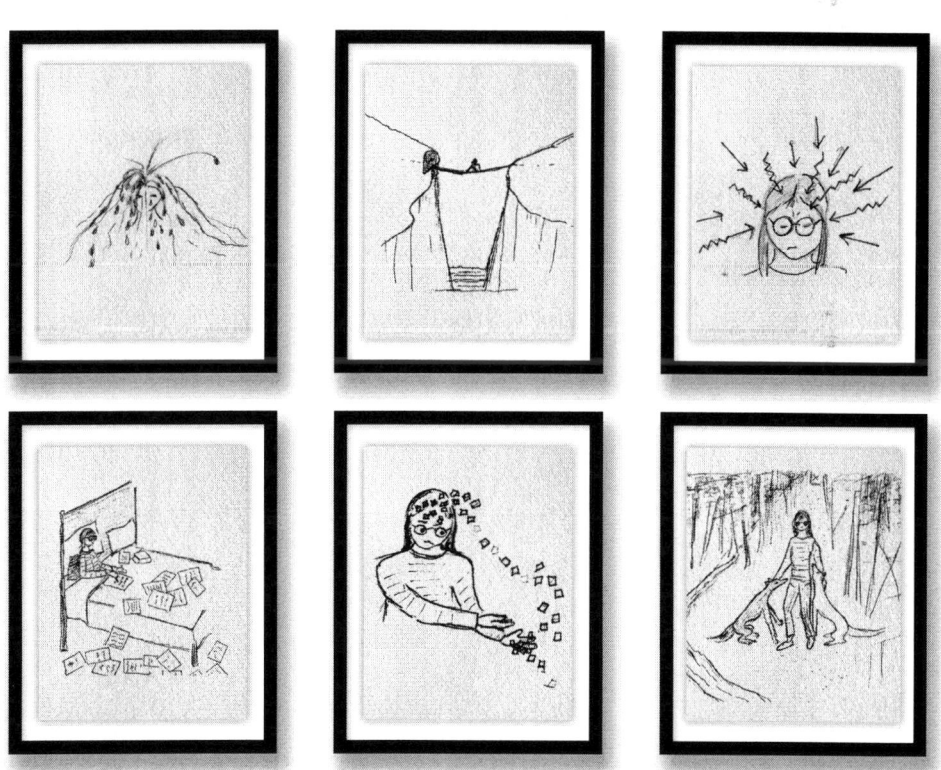

Chapter 13: Lightning Does Strike Twice

My life closed twice before its close
And it remains to see
If immortality unveil
A third event to me

So huge, so hopeless to conceive
As those that twice befell.
Parting is all we know of heaven
And all we need of hell.
(Emily Dickinson)

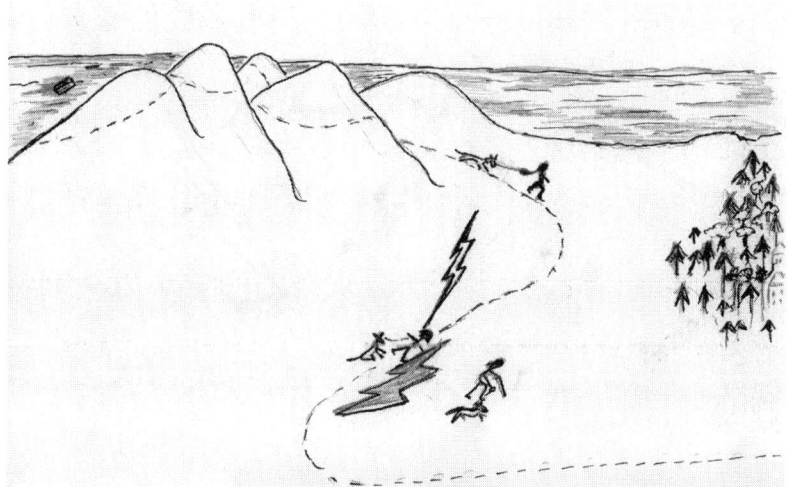

Finding my way down from the mountains

The going seems easier now. I am becoming accustomed. Getting up – doing all those things you need to do to get to work – slow, but there is a pattern… I have developed new ways of managing those simple – yet also complicated – tasks like getting up on time, dressing, making breakfast, getting to work.

I have all sorts of reminders and strategies to make sure I do things in the 'right' order and on time. Not that it ever goes smoothly. I can so easily get distracted – lose the sense of time. It is another of those areas where people say 'we all do that'. We do – but there seems to be an absoluteness for me now — whatever direction I go in, it is the only direction — so it is quite easy to completely forget I am going to work — or wherever it is that I am going. Before, I would still know somewhere in my mind that I was meant to be doing something else.

Also I knew what I was doing — I have notes — I had tasks written down and kept in view. I was learning that putting something in a file — in a drawer and closing it — could lead to forgetting it altogether.

So I was becoming adept at writing everything down — signposting to where next — before going to bed laying out the next day's tasks as I might lay out my clothes.

At last I really felt BACK. I enjoyed going in, holding meetings, teaching, getting a sense of the whole picture. I knew what we were doing, where we were going, what needed to be done.

The team had got used to me, I think — and would give me the prompts and reminders that I needed — so that the whole organising and planning within the Centre had an even stronger team sense than before.

We had had some team lunches out — I was beginning to be able to manage going into cafés — the noise of chatter and espresso machines and background music was still hard to filter out — but I was developing strategies, I was learning how to do this enough for it to be bearable, and to actually hear and follow what was being said!

The environment did continue to have all sorts of challenges however, so I liked to go to familiar places. This applied in work too and as long as I kept within a strong structure I could operate effectively, I felt.

I had also learnt to be more aware of my limits. For instance, a meeting or piece of work or planning, or going into a noisy environment could all tire me easily — my concentration would begin to go... and so I was learning to work within timescales that suited my needs.

I still felt very changed — I was very changed. I still would peer into the bathroom mirror at this face — these eyes — that were not mine — I feel I was making friends — becoming familiar with this me. As those around me became familiar too. This was just becoming that new normal.

Wedding preparations were in full swing. I had a Squirrel (instead of Hen) weekend to go to... I went down to Brighton again to buy my Mother-of-the-Bride hat. I could manage all of this — going out alone. Like a schoolchild proud to be managing without the grown-ups! I had to think about direction, draw myself maps of symbols to help me move around easily – limit my exposure to noise – cafes – too many decisions. But by pacing, planning, frequent stops... I could keep on track.

Now and then I did too much. It was still quite overwhelming to go into a restaurant and be with a group – the noise – the pace – the choices – what to eat. My brain still crashed. Particularly with certain background music.

And again – this was the new normal – instead of getting distressed as I had at first – I would pause – notice, breathe... ask for help if I needed it. I would often ask someone to come with me to somewhere I could recover – somewhere quieter. How kind and helpful people are. My family – my friends – my colleagues – unendingly supportive and understanding.

One of my dreads remained going to toilets in public buildings and cafés! Not unfamiliar from before the Haemorrhage – I imagine we must all have gone into toilets – particular the ones where there is a twisting route – up to another level or the ones in basements in cafés... in theatres, cinemas – and then wondered how to get out. Because I could no longer hold any sense of direction – or have any memory of which way I had come. I might manage one left turn and then another left or right (but this was advanced stuff!) but any more than that, and I would crash – with no idea which way to go. And wherever I turned at that point I would immediately forget which way it was – so was lost again. It was often quite scary.

I was home now in North Wales. It was only three weeks until the wedding. Excitement mounting – lots to do. I was looking forward to it so much. It was to be in a lovely venue – lots of family and friends from all over – I would take my puppy to play with the Lurcher owned by the family organising the event... Family were getting ready to travel up to North Wales.

I felt confident in what I had to do – I had written my Mother of the Bride speech. Things were going well in work. I went in for our monthly management meeting. For the first time since coming back I could actually remember who would be there, what our agenda was and what I wanted to bring up. The previous few meetings I had to read and be prompted – was not fully back into the work swing or be able to fully take on my role as Director, or of chairing meetings.

I remember driving in and noticing that driving too had become almost automatic again – I was back.

And then I discovered that lightning does strike twice. The meeting was halfway through, going smoothly – all the team were there – when I suddenly began to feel strange. There was a weird sensation in my head (different to the fizzings and buzzings left from the Haemorrhage and which had become familiar). I felt a lassitude – it was hard to focus my eyes – to sit up – and I was aware of a fear and a voice at the back of my brain protesting – No – No – you are fine – you cannot be ill – don't let this happen – keep going. I knew – could observe that something was going wrong in my head – but the determination not to give in to it was so strong – No No not again – this cannot happen again – fighting – I could see that others were noticing something was wrong – a voice said 'are you okay Jody?' – I think I said Yes, I don't know, my face felt funny – voices came from far away and then I felt myself keel over to the side. For a brief moment I think I lost consciousness. And then I was lying down on a couch – just trying to get up – to carry on – NO NO NO – I knew where I was – I knew what WAS HAPPENING – I knew the wedding was near – this couldn't happen now. I was chairing this meeting – I can't be lying down, I have to hold it all together – for them… this was my job… then for my family I was afraid – afraid it was the same again – that I would go again into that other post-haemorrhage world – or maybe this time die. I was needed – No, not now. I could not go now – I was needed for the wedding… My daughter needed me – I could not be ill now…

I am not sure what was happening – but that there was discussion around me about what to do – and I think they had called an ambulance. I tried to sit up. I wasn't unconscious – I managed to speak… I was fine – I would be fine in a moment. But everyone was insistent that I needed to go to hospital.

I wanted to stay – I needed to carry on holding the meeting, I thought – to make sure everybody was all right – assure them that all would be okay… this seemed awful. My last Haemorrhage had been on my own – I found it harder to be among others – for them to witness that and wonder how that was for them… plus being angry – determined to be okay in a minute. I would NOT go to hospital.

It is all so clear in my mind. Surprising, because so much else isn't. It stands out – like some events do – in my memory now. As if a spotlight is shining on it.

It was only two weeks to the wedding – I couldn't be ill – how would that affect everything – the plans. It would upset everything – I was fighting. But of course – there was nothing I could do. I felt quite helpless.

I remember the ambulance journey – then being in the hospital in Bangor – later transferred back to Walton. I do not often get despairing – but those were terrible moments. This was not just about ME now – and of course it wasn't before. But I wanted the wedding to all be lovely – as you do – my Daughter – what would happen – would they have to postpone – all the chaos of that – the disappointment – would they carry on without me… how would that be – I would be ruining everything…

But this was not what I had had before. It was not the coiling in my brain leaking so that the blood from the aneurysm burst out – I did not need an operation. This was a haemorrhage but a different sort… a subdural haemorrhage. There had been bleeding into my brain, but slow bleeding, and the blood had built up and pressed on the brain resulting in this Stroke – that was why I was conscious – it was not the same as before. The blood was gradually being absorbed – this is a very unmedical description of what I understood of what was happening.

I was only in hospital for perhaps four days then I was able to come home.

It didn't seem to have affected me that much – except that I was more tired. We were all so relieved. Now I could just get back to how things were before that fateful meeting.

But it wasn't to be quite that straightforward. This Haemorrhage carried its own set of consequences and changes. But for now I was at home. Tired, quite easily confused, I would need some support over the wedding weekend – but all was going ahead.

The consequences would gradually reveal themselves as the years rolled on.

Chapter 14: The Landscape Changes

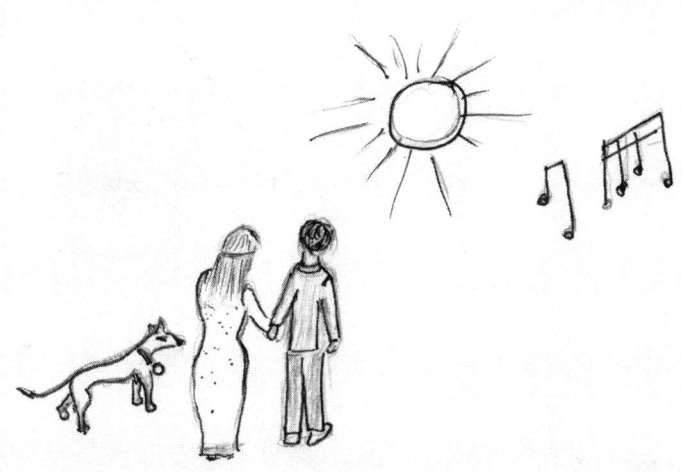

Despite the upheaval and uncertainty around me in those crucial two weeks leading up to the first Wedding, we were all able to pick up the threads, and plans continued – work agendas and wedding preparations happening in tandem.

We were all carrying on almost as if nothing had happened, and I think that added to the sense of unreality for me. I was still reeling from the 'lightning strike' but I was 'OK' – just let's get on with things now – 'thank goodness it wasn't serious'. And so I carried on, to some degree on a sort of auto-pilot, a denial that anything much had happened.

It was a Wonderful Wedding – many families and friends – all coming together on one of those Golden Summer Days that seemed familiar to me from long ago – a sense of Childhood – a long day with nothing but pleasure.

Everything looked so beautiful – all D and C's planning – the wonderful flowers (including masses of sweet peas on the round table for the Wedding Tea – actually grown by me in my garden – with the help of my friend Heather who was also doing all the Wedding flowers – and probably the first flowers I have ever managed to grow successfully!)

And I even managed to stand up and make my speech! I was so pleased – I had so wanted to do that for my daughter – to celebrate her and welcome C. I had to read it – but I WAS there.

It was a flawless day – the weather – the guests – the house – the ceremony – the food. I think there was great relief all round that it was happening and that I was well – that wonderful kindness and good will from so many people – my wonderful family – and over and over again great waves of relief – it could so easily have been different.

And yet for me – and I hoped only for me – that no one else saw – I knew I was only half there – I felt like a ghost walking among the crowd and the flowers and the laughter – there but not quite there. Something in me had changed – I didn't know then what it was – but there was a subtle difference in how people looked – how I was able to relate to them. That wonderful sense of connection to people that had been a gift I felt from the first Haemorrhage – had changed – except with my family – and those people I knew very well – I felt invisible.

Before, my organisation of time had not been too good – but now I had the first hints of new changes – I very quickly lost awareness of what I was meant to be doing – oh – tea now… oh – the ceremony now – someone would come and make sure I was in the right place.

I remember being aware of this – and not liking it – something felt wrong. I should be doing this – supporting D and C – as well as their wonderful Best Man and Bridesmaid and friends and the rest of our family – but I wasn't. I was not the Me I had always been – even since the First Bleed. I felt stunned – would just stand or sit – letting others do things – make decisions. Unless there was something specific I had to do (like making the speech) I just didn't seem to do anything.

I missed the first group photo – I had wandered off – quite unaware of what was going on – everyone was calling me apparently – it was a while before I heard them and joined the group for the rest of the photos. This was so unlike me. I knew it but it was almost as if I was in a dream.

D and C have that first photo – the large group gathered together on the Porch with a gap – beside D – a gap where I should have been, and then, in the other photos I am there… standing among them all. But it is not quite me – a ghost of me.

It was only some years later that I realised how that sense of not being quite there – WITH people – IN the world, almost a ghost walking among them because I could not be seen as the me I am now… became clear to me.

And there were changes from that second Brain Haemorrhage – mostly unnoticed by others and disregarded because 'it was not serious'. I think it was some years before even those close to me began to see that. I remember the relief when someone said, 'things did change after that second bleed didn't they... I didn't realise it then'.

And the main thing was, of course, I WAS there... I AM here... and it is just that there were more changes that arose from that Subdural bleed. Not so obvious, but nevertheless they have remained. They of course became a part of my journey. And that means everyone who I am connected to – it has become part of their journey to some extent or other.

Is this the consequence of all illness and injury? Certainly of those that are life changing – anything life changing is going to impact on others too.

I went into quite a different phase after this. My map of my journey... The journey that had started a year ago on 5 August with the Tsunami in my Brain – continued down to the cliffs and the great abyss of the sea far below. Painfully and slowly I am traversing a thin rope bridge suspended high over the waves... leaning on my stick.

Step by step leaving behind my old familiar world – the gate to that world was shut now – I could not go that way again. I could only go forward. One step at a time – this breath, this breath. And then stepping out on the new land – huge rolling heathland into the distance. Mountains showing way up ahead. And that slow walk, this step – this step – until at last I reach the mountains – back to work – my puppy – driving – climbing the foothills – struggling through the peaks – and finally the easier descent on to the plains... and back to work...

And then the Lightning strike of the Second Bleed – lying by an abyss – I could see the depths again – but I got up and was there at the Wedding – like arriving at a shining city along the way.

And now I was up and walking again – back to work.

Perhaps we all thought that I would just carry on now – that word Recovery – I would get better and better.

Most of the difficult things left over from my time off before had now been ironed out. My life at home was largely organised; I had help where I needed it. I was working with my Neuropsychologist – cognitive testing, talking, I had somewhere to explore the changes, understand them and talk through the difficulties they brought.

Chapter 14: The Landscape Changes

D and C were on their honeymoon and then returned to their lives – F and K were now preparing for their Wedding and later there would a birth. I had my nieces and great nieces visiting me – friends – my puppy – it was a wonderful and hopeful time. And yet I was still learning how to be. There were constant internal shifts between a warm connected sense of being present and then just turning a corner that might take me into quite a different place – confused – unsure – time has slipped – what am I doing – why am I here.

Noticing... Balancing... disguising – trying to be something I had not read about yet.

I had that sense that this was how it was meant to be... After Brain haemorrhages – and that I should be living up to this in some way. I needed to really get 'better' now – just get on with it...

And yet now, for the first time I began to feel ashamed, and to hide. I was not the same. It was not all OK. I was not at all sure I could manage. I didn't really understand what was going on for me, even though I am a Mindfulness Teacher, a Psychotherapist and I had such supportive friends who knew about these things. As Director of the Centre for Mindfulness, I felt I should be more aware and in control – I had begun to gather it all together – and to some degree that continued – I could see the direction – I did know what I needed to do within the Team and in my role in the University – that overall picture which had been so missing when I first came back to work a year ago after the first bleed.

And I had so much help and support from friends and colleagues – Cognitive Testing and Support and support from the University. And I was working with Frances who is contributing to this book – a friend and colleague and Neuropsychologist with a wide knowledge of Brain Injury and Mindfulness.

Frances came to see me and listened – listened to my long, probably rambling accounts of how it was to be me... and she understood what I was saying and explained it to me in neurological and psychological terms that I could understand.

It is what we are writing about here. Everything I experience, as for all of us – coloured by the people we are, seen through the lens of our own lives – childhood, experiences that form who we are and how we see ourselves and how we build and manage relationships. How we live and die.

Yet my landscape had changed again. My headaches had become more frequent and more severe again.

I once again needed to rely on a stick – I found it hard to walk very far and quickly tired.

I had to be aware of temperature – in a way I had never accounted before – I got cold or easily overheated. There was a lot of looking at my blood pressure – monitoring it.

The fizzing in my head – sudden sharp lightning pains – and strange sensations were quite intense again.

I was both very fatigued and had trouble sleeping.

And, for the first time, I began to feel uneasy in company – I had lost some confidence, I think. In myself – and I had become distrustful of others, sure that they must be finding me a nuisance. *Did they think I was putting it on? Making a fuss.*

I seemed to be walking in a lonely place – behind me the mountains – and in front I could only see a dark forest.

And I returned to my Mindfulness Practice – settling, grounding and sitting watching my breath, seeing if I could allow all the difficulties to just be here. I knew – from my reading and experience – that when we want things to be different – when we want to get rid of them and push them away – actually they just get stronger.

This is a hard practice – having an intention to Accept pain, discomfort and difficulty – and now, because my mood was low – it was even harder.

I found it helpful to do short Walking Meditations.

Chapter 15: The Edge of the Woods

A Road Through the Woods
Two roads diverged in a yellow wood,
And sorry I could not travel both
And be one traveller, long I stood
And looked down one as far as I could
To where it bent in the undergrowth;

Then took the other, as just as fair,
And having perhaps the better claim,
Because it was grassy and wanted wear;
Though as for that the passing there
Had worn them really about the same,

And both that morning equally lay
In leaves no step had trodden black.
Oh, I kept the first for another day!
Yet knowing how way leads on to way,
I doubted if I should ever come back.

I shall be telling this with a sigh
Somewhere ages and ages hence:
Two roads diverged in a wood, and I –
I took the one less travelled by,
And that has made the difference.
(Robert Frost)

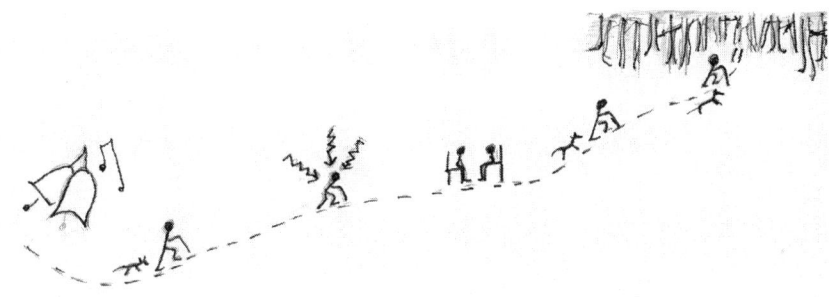

Chapter 15: The Edge of the Woods

The path through the woods was a long path. The sense of being in the woods came from feeling quite confined – shapes seemed to loom around and beside me – dark – just out of vision. I would very determinedly put one foot at a time on the path ahead – whatever was happening with my eyes – but this meant that I had to turn my head to see anything that was not directly in front of me. There was no going back. The only thing I could do was to go on. To experience whatever was there to be experienced. There was no hiding because what I was hiding from was in my head.

In a way it had been like that since the beginning – I just put one foot in front of the other and looked ahead. But this time, after the second Bleed and the first wedding, it seemed different. It is hard to explain – things just looked and felt different. The things that had been a struggle before – organising time – awareness of where objects were on my desk – keeping track of time itself and being where I needed to be – all this somehow felt fuzzy – and took a lot of effort. Effort, that is what I remember – if I took my attention away from something for long then it was as if it disappeared. I might be reading something – or in the middle of a series of email conversations – but I knew I was not following through the threads. I had a constant sense of things falling away. And this looming sense of darkness.

On the surface, presumably I did not look any different to anyone. This had not been a 'serious bleed' – I needed no surgery – I returned to work quite soon. Whatever had happened to me was invisible. So this was a lonely path. I also did not want to 'make a fuss' – upset people – so I began to pretend that everything was all right – surely it was? This was just me. Looking back now it is hard to explain – so I think I will just tell 'the stories'.

I became overwhelmed by the amount of THINGS around me – in my house – bookshelves – all the objects, the kitchen – cupboards full of things – all the belongings that make up our personal space. Most of it felt irrelevant. I could not remember what was IN anything – things in boxes or cupboards simply did not exist. Most of it seemed to belong to someone else. Too many things on display and they started to move – crowding my vision. I started two processes – one was to put lots of things previously on display away in cupboards – and to put anything I knew I wanted to use out where I could see it clearly. I moved so many things that I did not know where anything was. Eventually this led to me having my whole house painted indoors with the same very light colour. I was not comfortable with the amount of different colours I had before, each room a different shade. Now everything off-white.

I had my family and dear friends and a new wonderful neighbour who agreed to clean for me. Together we filled up endless huge boxes of THINGS – and I sent them all away. I had always had a lot of paintings and photos on my walls – now I had just a few. It probably doesn't sound too important – but it was this different person – I was finding out what she liked – I could not live comfortably in my old environment. My old life had been on display with colour schemes that did not belong to the ME I am now. That seemed like a strange thing – many things that I had previously liked I no longer did. Everything had to be uncluttered, simple, spaced.

And it was around this time that the HUM arrived. I just noticed one day that there was this loud HUM in the house – I spent a lot of time trying to work out where it came from – no one else could hear it. That was so upsetting because it was there all the time. Going to sleep became hard – when I lay down to try to sleep all I could hear was the Hum. I was convinced at first that it was electrical – but then realised that it was with me wherever I was – out for walks – maybe it was the electric pylons? When I went into other houses and buildings – there it was... the HUM. I started to wonder if the Brain Haemorrhages had done something to my brain that made me very sensitive to hearing electrical currents or something. I went to see the Doctor and was referred to a Tinnitus specialist. She said this was not Tinnitus but some of the things that helped with Tinnitus could help me. This helped me to realise that this WAS ME – not something outside of me – but my experience was as if I was hearing something from outside. I think the idea that it was IN me was terrifying. Would I have to live with this forever? Could I bear it? I knew too that I was probably boring everyone with it – so I began to go inward, I felt trapped, nothing much was here except me and the HUM.

But I carried on. I was back in work (accompanied by the HUM). It was more manageable when I was doing other things. The worst times were at night – trying to read quietly or to sleep...

I felt strange at work around this time. Coming back after the Wedding and the Second Haemorrhage – I was able to pick up the pieces – My sense of the whole of the Agency – meetings and my ideas around what needed to be developed – they were all there. I found some refuge in putting my attention into this. But trying to actually DO what was needed – emailing – typing documents – following through – remembering where anything was filed – all this took a great deal of effort and attention. I could clearly see an overall plan – what needed to happen where – but following it through was a different matter. I seemed to have difficulty in moving from the whole vision to part of the vision. Later, I thought it was rather like watching a film. You know it is the whole film – the whole story – but can only see that one scene at a time – all the rest is out of sight.

I could manage quite well if I was just on my own – but if someone came in and talked to me, phoned me – then that could take my attention completely into responding to THAT. I seemed to fall from one thing to another – leaving behind a trail of unfinished tasks – as I tumbled into a new one.

I would sit at my desk and get everything organised – I needed to have just a few things set out to do. I needed complete quiet and no interruptions. Then I would make a list of what needed to be done for each of those things. I would write it all down. I learnt that I could manage to hold perhaps three or four things at the most – depending on how tired I was – but any more and the whole thing would collapse.

I went back to my way of separating tasks – there were ORANGES tasks – so I put them in a Bowl – then there were other tasks – and they went in a different bowl – APPLES – they were not so important. It was the oranges that I had to do first.

And I would sit down very focused on each orange – knowing just what had to be done… maybe a paper to write – or a phone call to make – an email to send – some filing to do – a course programme to design – the minutes of a meeting to dictate. The strange thing was that I COULD DO ALL THESE THINGS – but if someone came in and in any way disturbed me – put a message on the desk – said 'just let me tell you about'… everything would go. It was as if the oranges fell out of the bowl and all rolled around on the floor.

And my head would simply empty – no memory of what I was doing – where I was. It is a terrible feeling – nowhere to go – no idea where I had come from – just a space of confusion and blankness, and underneath it was fear – knowing something was wrong – but not knowing how to get back. I could feel the space where the information had been before my attention was taken away from it. Sometimes I could almost see it trickling away – trying to grasp it was like trying to grasp water. Or I would feel the GAP as something had just fallen off a cliff. Gone. Sometimes of course, things came back – although not quite in the same way. I learnt I just had to Trust and be prepared to let go. If I tried to grasp – search for the lost memory, that seemed to push it even further away.

This was a lonely time. I didn't feel I could talk about this. I was meant to be 'in charge', to 'know what I was doing'. It felt very shameful to be so 'incompetent' – and I began to really doubt myself. Interestingly, I was fine in meetings – face to face with people. I could teach and give a talk – chair a meeting – but not manage the written word, and filing was particularly difficult – putting things in the right places.

To some extent I had enough insight to see what I was doing. Frances helped me to reflect and begin to get an overall view of what was going on for me. What was wonderful was that she was so accepting. She was interested in what was happening to me, and never once gave me the idea it was 'wrong' or that I should learn to be different. She normalised it all in terms of, 'this is what happens when you have a Sub Arachnoid Haemorrhage'. This was such a relief. I didn't have to pretend anything. I could say 'I am afraid' – 'I don't remember' – 'I don't think I am organising things well enough'.

And she named and explained the processes I was using to manage – like the oranges. She even told me that it was clever of me to notice what was happening!

I learnt from this how little people, even colleagues in the University, know about Brain Injury and the business of losing memory. So many times people have either minimised it – 'oh, we all do that, sometimes you just need to be more organised'. Some people – so kindly meant – gave me books on how to be organised. They were full of tables and boxes of what to do, which left me feeling almost dizzy and confused. What I found I needed was more SPACE, not to fill up what was there with systems.

Chapter 16: Leaving Work and the Hum in the Woods

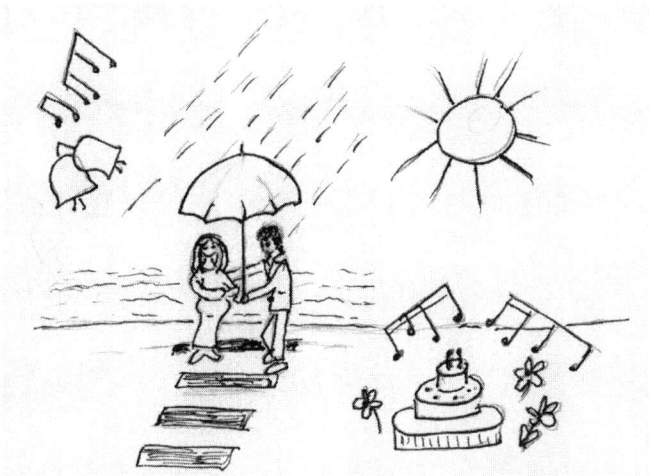

As the Summer of 2011 came to an end, it was time for F and K's Wedding – another wonderful family time. K and F were celebrating their marriage and the years they had already spent together bringing up R, who was there as Best Man.

It was some months since my second Haemorrhage and I was much more present and able to participate fully – although by now – in the background – there was always 'the Hum'.

Images from the day stay with me. Us all in the rather grand Llandudno Town Hall. K beautiful in her white dress and very pregnant. F in his suit and R as Best Man. Outside it was raining and we waved them off from the Registry Office in the Land Rover. There is a wonderful picture of F holding a huge umbrella over K as they crossed the Zebra Crossing to the George Hotel with a stormy sea in the background… inside so beautifully arranged and warm with family and friends. And later our close family drove to Pwllheli to stay in a Hotel and we all had a wonderful and beautifully decorated family meal. I remember feeling overwhelmed by the happiness of it all – after the ups and downs of the last year – my two Haemorrhages – D and C's wonderful wedding in the summer and now F and K's wedding two months later with their baby on the way. And I was well – I was there – I felt that somehow we had all come through some dangerous territory and now the sun had come out.

For a few months everything went back to normal. D and C went back to Brighton – I was back at work and trying to pick up the pieces again… and then it was nearly Christmas and K went into Labour. D and C drove up – and our A was born on 11 December. I knew I could easily not have been here.
It had been an extraordinary year.

And as we moved into the next year, everyone went back again into their normal lives – and A became a part of us, as children do.

But as we moved into everyday life, I had the sense of things closing in around me. I was different after this second haemorrhage. It was nothing dramatic, and I tried to hide it from my family, for I felt they had all had enough. But I knew I was different – my sense of space – of the space around me, had changed. I often felt as if the walls were falling towards me, falling in on me – things moved in the corners of my vision. My headaches were bad – in a way I was used to them, they were part of life, but nevertheless unpleasant – unrelenting. I went to sleep to them and woke up to them. I used my practice – I knew I needed to Accept they were there. I did not have to like them, but when I wanted them to go away, I gave more attention to them and they seemed to get stronger.

And the Hum, that noise, also grew stronger and more persistent. I tried not to think about it, but the more I tried not to, the more I was aware of the humming. I became obsessed with trying to find the source. It seemed to be everywhere and nowhere. My head itself was 'noisy'. There were clicking noises and often that familiar fizzing sensation – and now I could even HEAR the fizzing sound too. That meant I stayed focused on it – and it was exhausting – it was hard to rest – to sleep – even to go out and walk – everything was accompanied by the Hum.

Looking back, I think a lot of this may have been me adjusting to all the changes. In a way I think I was still in shock from the second Haemorrhage – because 'nothing had happened' – there was no brain injury – everything went on as normal and it was ignored – but it had been something – something HAD happened. I was learning a little more about what Brain Injury means. To a large degree it is EXPERIENCED – not something others can see – or even begin to understand. It is a lonely place.

But I was getting used to it – it had just taken a while for me to adjust to this – yet again – new me. It was nowhere near as dramatic as the First Haemorrhage – the new eyes and the loss of self – but that was all still there. The perceptual changes that had been there from the first journey home in the car from the Hospital – were magnified now by the subtle changes in perception that came with the second Haemorrhage. It wasn't going to go away, or get better. Perhaps it was permanent. That was frightening.

It is hard to describe these sorts of experiences to others – I think we often need to have experienced something similar to be able to understand others' experiences.

I had my Mindfulness Practice – and that helped me settle when my head was noisy and painful – to breathe and be grounded – and to allow and accept that this was just the way things were. I sought to accept whatever was here.

It was still strange to go into work as if nothing had happened. I was finding it even harder to organise things – the constant noise in my head was so distracting... But I was determined to carry on. I had a clear plan of action, and I tried so hard to ignore it all.

In the end, of course, that was just exhausting. I would go into work, make my list of what needed attending to – making sure, as I had learnt to, that I only had a maximum of three tasks on the table. Of course, as the day went on, more tasks built up. The bowl soon overflowed with oranges – and eventually they would all tumble onto the floor – lost – and I would have to stop – rest a while, then hopefully be able to pick some of them up.

I knew I couldn't go on.

At this time it began to seem as if I was walking in a dark wood. There were trees close around me – and not much light came in through the leaves. It was hard to find my way around in this new world.

I think I knew that my old life was behind me now – and the Hum, that humming noise that had been there for a while, got much louder and more persistent. It was there all the time – driving to work, at work, at home, when I tried to go to sleep. Strangely, I carried on – I still had my overall plan and picture of what I wanted at work, for the team. We were all meeting, planning, taking the Centre forward – the work was getting done. But it was very frustrating. On one level I could see all this. I had a sense of my team and what they needed, the Teachers, the wider team – but the noise was getting louder – drowning things out. I knew it was getting harder to hold it all. I was relying so much on my wonderful Office Manager and my team.

Everything got muddled, at home and at work – now I could not put anything away – once something was put in a file or a drawer then it ceased to exist – it would never come out again. I gradually became surrounded by paper – lists – books. Everything was out and piled up – I think it contributed to the sense of walking in a wood – a narrow path with things piled up, bushes and trees, on either side.

I realised that I could not continue to work as Director. The realisation had come slowly but now I was quite sure – and since then, there have been so many things – so many roles to let go of. It is hard to describe the sensation in my head as I tried to gather up all the things that have to be remembered and carried over day by day. Before it had been so easy – but no more. Each day I would try to gather up all the thoughts, plans, knowledge… things long known as well as newly acquired but they would all tumble together, like balls gradually rolling down a slope and then over an edge – I could see them – reach out – but never grasp them. They were gone, lying in a heap somewhere.

We don't realise we are doing it – this out of awareness filing that we do moment by moment through our days. What we have done – the memories – what we are going to do next – what that will lead to in the long term… we hold so much.

I didn't quite understand what was happening to me back then. Now I am looking back some years later and I am more familiar with the 'crashes' and the tumbling away of thoughts, plans, structures, memories – short and long term. It happens most days – and that is the territory of my Brain Injury.

Now I can stand in the midst of the tumbling thoughts, there is a sensation in my head as they fall – a bit nauseous – and I just let them go. Fighting it makes it worse and leads to regret and suffering. At least I have learnt not to do that anymore. I have a ritual now as I see something go – I thank it for having visited me and wish it well. I notice the difference in my heart and body when I do that. I have a choice – to grasp and regret and feel miserable – or to be grateful for what I have had and wish it well. There is more contentment that way.

I know that sooner or later my head will settle down. Sometimes I may even be able to pick up some of the pieces and carry on. It is as if the picture that I hold in my head – of who I am and what I am doing – suddenly cracks apart and becomes a Jigsaw puzzle. Some days I can move some of the pieces. Other times, I just pack them away in a box.

Sometimes there is someone there to help, but mostly it is a lonely place. People soon realise that this is a never ending Jigsaw Puzzle and they quietly move away. There is no 'getting better', 'being as before' – there is only the repeated Puzzle. At first I was sad at that, but now I understand. We are on different paths – have different ways of thinking and seeing the world. Even if we make the Jigsaw Puzzle, it is NOT the same as the picture of life before – it has cracks all through it. This is MY path – and I believe it has been my Mindfulness practice that has helped me accept that.

Neuro Notes 4: New Challenges

As recovery continues in the months and years after a stroke or brain injury, life is likely to throw up new challenges, just as it did before the injury. For example, moving house, going back to work, another illness, a bereavement or a separation.

New challenges and life events can bring to light difficulties that were not recognised before. Extra stress can also aggravate physical health problems, as well as memory and concentration difficulties. The person may feel they are going backwards rather than getting better, even if they were coping well before things changed. Adapting to change often takes longer and requires more effort than it did before the stroke.

Jody's second brain haemorrhage had far-reaching consequences, despite being less serious than the first. She was more aware of her difficulties, and her mood was lower. People are more susceptible to depression after a stroke or brain injury, especially when they become aware of their losses.

The person may feel that they should be able to cope better, or feel guilty about being a 'burden' on others. They may feel ashamed or embarrassed, see their situation as hopeless, or feel helpless and may want to give up.

People often feel more anxious than usual when new challenges arise. The person may believe that they cannot cope, and want to hide away. It is important to do as much as possible, build confidence, and stay in contact with people, and to have enough support to be able to do this.

It can be helpful to notice negative thoughts about difficulties, and to recognise signs of anxiety. Butterflies in the tummy, constant worrying, feeling panicky, and feeling clammy or short of breath are common signs of anxiety.

Being aware of our thoughts – as simply thoughts and not facts – and recognising the body sensations involved in fear and anxiety takes away some of their power. Try to let the thoughts and feelings go, as though they are dark clouds passing across the sky. Being caught up in them tends to make mood lower, and anxiety worse.

Focus on something that is happening around you instead, or on your breathing. Listen to music or a relaxation recording, or do some physical exercise. Paying attention to something else will help at the time. Talk to someone else about how you are feeling.

Part 5: Into the Woods

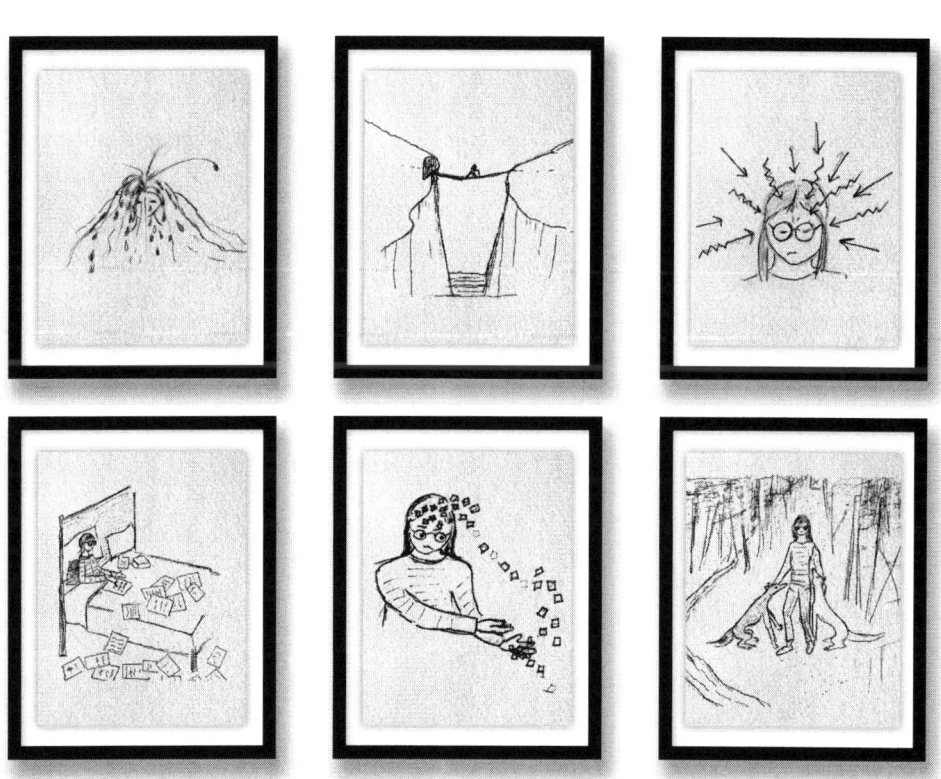

Chapter 17: Further into the Woods

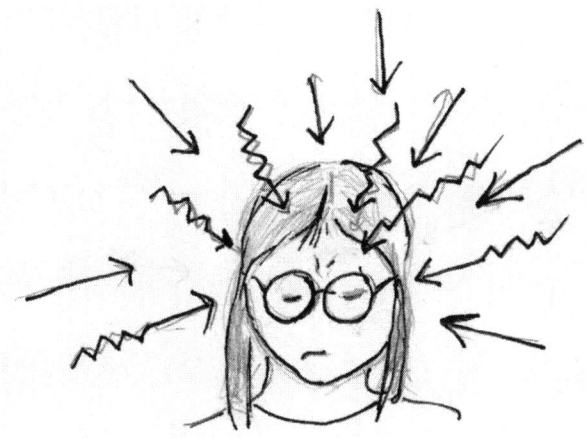

Some things seemed to be getting harder. I had thought, perhaps, things would get back to being more normal – forgetting perhaps that there was no familiar normal – only NEW NORMAL.

The Oranges were still slipping off the table – as I actually became quicker and able to do more, at the same time there was more to crash out of my memory.

Overall I did seem to see what was needed – have overall plans – but at the same time I was not able to split the whole into smaller chunks – different tasks. As soon as I did that – off they would roll into that pile of muddled things forgotten or waiting to be sorted. I became anxious about being seen as not managing. I felt I should be doing 'Better' by now – I was quite judgemental of myself – and paranoid about what others might be thinking. The result of all this was that I began to feel more isolated – that I was a drain and drowning – that I just couldn't do it all.

I could teach a mindfulness course, a session on the Masters course. But these are contained sessions. I could not organise things – pull together several strands to make a whole. They seemed to be very different tasks with needs for different strengths.

All this contributed in the end to deciding to leave my role as Director of the Mindfulness Centre. I was just going to keep my role of occasional teacher, trainer and supervisor. It was both a relief and a great sadness.

I felt quite lost. Who and what was I? For the first time I realised I was cut off in the middle of something – my life direction.

Gradually I seemed to have left a lot of the structures of my previous life.

As well as being Director of the Centre, I had also been a Mindfulness Teacher and Trainer for many years. Although no longer active, I was a qualified Psychotherapist who had a thriving private practice and a role as trainer of Psychotherapists in three different Training Institutes. All this had gone – I couldn't even remember those theories I had known so well – taken so long to learn… and yet – I could work in a different way with people – with mindfulness and with the immediacy of being with someone. I could use mindfulness with a therapeutic intention – but I could not be a Psychotherapist.

Gradually I was realising that I did not want to hold all those activities I used to know so well – I began to acknowledge how much had been washed away with my Haemorrhages. And that I did not have the energy or the capacity to learn it all again.

At this time my Mindfulness practice too, which had so sustained me, seemed less deep, less regular. I had been part of several groups – as a Mindfulness teacher – as a trainer – as a Psychotherapist – regular monthly meetings with dear colleagues and friends – and all of this too had gone. And what was left, I had to let go.

I could not travel far – nor drive for an hour or more to a meeting and then back again. I didn't know how.

It is not easy to explain Brain Injury – and I don't think I understood what it really meant for me until then.

Every journey I undertook needed to be on a very well-known route. I could not easily remember any new direction – if at all – and could no longer follow directions or use a Sat Nav – previously my saviour.

In fact, the Sat Nav caused me some pretty confused moments until I realised what was happening and turned it off. When you get to a turning, or roundabout – it says 'Turn left'. That was fine. I could remember to turn left – but almost as soon as it has said 'Turn left', it gives another instruction… 'and then Turn right'. My brain immediately crashed. Two instructions close together – this is one of the things I still cannot do – and this was extremely distressing because

I did not understand what was happening. This experience of being given more than one option – or one piece of information… It is the bowl of oranges again. Even now – writing a long time later and very familiar with this – everything has to be One at a Time. Now, too, I understand enough to explain to others – back then, it was just all confusion and distress – and when it came to driving… fear. And it was not long before I gave up anything but totally familiar and short journeys. Always in the daytime – the night light reflection blinded and distracted me.

And back to the meetings – I could no longer sit through a long meeting – and also I would not remember any of the content. I did remember the connection and contact with others though – that was, and has been, the greatest loss and sadness. The people. And of course I did lose contact. It is not easy to explain Brain Injury – so I felt my actions were probably often misunderstood.

The picture in my mind of this time is of me walking onto a path through some woods. I seemed alone and also had a sense of going forward, but there seemed to be lots of obstacles just at the edge of my vision – and also there was still, and growing louder, the Hum.

I think that contributed to this sense that I was among trees – and the Hum was the noise of the wood – and nothing and no one seemed to be around – mostly anyway. And somehow that was easier – I didn't have to explain anything – I couldn't get anything wrong for anyone – I could just do what I do. And that was stopping and sitting on my cushion and meditating – or walking one step at a time. Learning to focus my attention, to bring my attention in from the chaos that was in my head to just one point. The Breath and the Body sitting or walking. And also to an attitude of Kindness – towards everything around me, towards my dear family and friends who were having to support me and deal with what to me seemed like chaos – and to myself. It was all too easy to be critical and cross with myself – as I think I would have been without a mindfulness practice and this way of looking at things. And Kindness. Breathing in Kindness to myself, Breathing out kindness to others.

But I was lost. I didn't know where I was going. I was lonely because I was somehow not the same with people any more. We were all getting used to the changes in me. I was lonely because I had lost a familiar part of me – and memories – some memories came back – but some may well be gone for ever. I also seemed to have forgotten bits of how I look after myself – organise myself.

The Hum had become louder – and more constant – more insistent. Listen to me. Listen to me. Struggling to hear and not to hear the hum – what is it – where is it? Always seemed just out of reach – I saw it as outside me – and later struggled against the idea that it was me.

I tried to get free of it – it was in my house – I was feeling overwhelmed by everything, even my home and garden seemed too big – had too many things in it – too much colour. And I wanted desperately to get away from it.

A friend who managed a Caravan Park close by helped me hire a Caravan. It was not summer – and there were very few people there. I loved it – my family helped by taking food and a few things up there – and I and my dog moved into our new, compact home. Quiet – with the box of food, I didn't even have to shop. I just had my radio – my painting things – and a notebook and pencil.

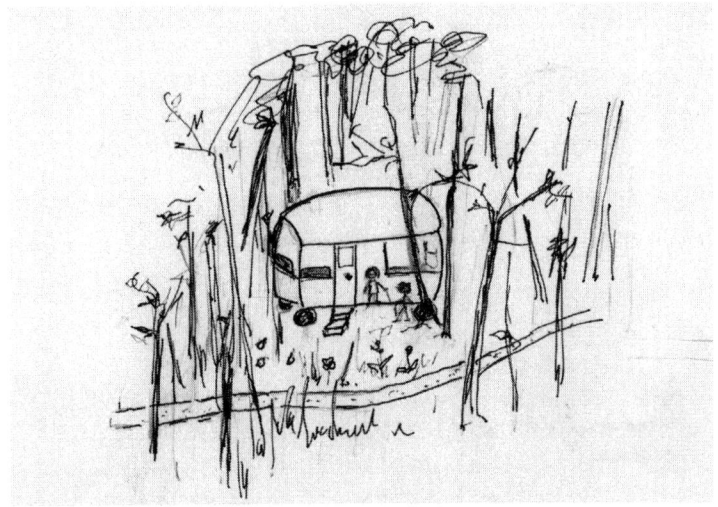

Chapter 18: Wolves in the Woods

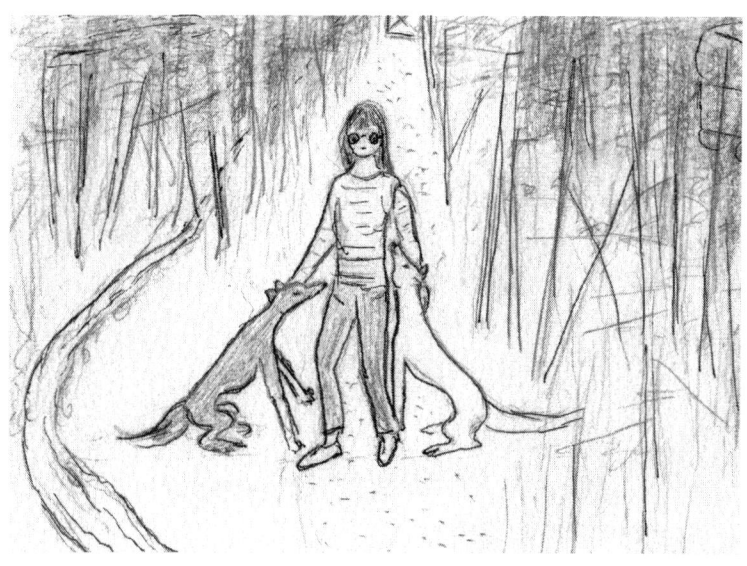

No Compass

Where do we go from here?
What is beyond?
Not knowing, I am fearful
and ask for certainty or at least a compass
to solid ground.

There is a station existing between two tunnels
You must travel through darkness to arrive there.
Keep along the tracks when the sun goes down
carrying all you can. No straight line to awareness
The only currency is kindness.

What is beyond imagining?
Summer in midwinter
Snow on a hot June day.
God in heaven.
No solid ground.

Chapter 18: Wolves in the Woods

What is beyond bearing?
A world without you.
The death of a child.
Leaving home…

The sun is weak in January but you will be safe in the woods.
Some call them the dark woods. The moss is a carpet of stars
clothing the trunks of trees. alongside ivy and lichen.
There are no wolves only foxes.

When you stumble on the stream follow it by sound
to the river and all the way to the sea.

I am determined to stay on the path.
Alone in a strange country
Beyond sun and shadow

With no compass.
(Annee Griffiths)

In many ways I am getting on with normal life – well, as normal as it can be. I am managing life – shopping, driving, organising what I do to some extent – seeing my family – friends – being this person they all see and experience and being this person they do not see. And despite the normality of all this, I feel I am being almost herded deeper into the woods.

I have a sense of a twilight around me – at the edges of my vision great trees rise up into the sky – I see the path ahead – it is not always clear, covered with leaves, muddy, sandy – but the trees part to allow the path to be there. I follow it – I can hear the quiet and the movement of the trees – sometimes wind and leaves rustling and that makes me aware of the Humming that is always there in my head… I notice it – allow it to be there. But there are not many leaves, it must be winter. Many of the trees are dark, black – something whispers – deeper in – deeper in… I can see the path ahead – I know somewhere if I just keep going I will come to a Gate – I have to get there, my way lies through it.

For a while I have been aware of how I can move between thoughts that are distressing, threatening, full of fear and anxiety at what may happen, and also thoughts of kindness, soothing, reassurance. My practice – my Mindfulness again so helpful here, I can just sit with what I do not like and fear and what I want and am attracted to.

And as I walk in the woods I seem to see dark movements at the edge of my vision – and I know they are Wolves – they are familiar, I have met them many times before — they are here with me – accompanying me on my journey.

I remember the story that we all have our own wolves: 'The Wolf of Love and the Wolf of Hate'. They are often present in us through our lives and sometimes they speak to us. The Wolf of Hate invites us to hate – to want to get rid of things, to doubt, for things to be different – to fight against and push away what we don't want. The Wolf of Love invites us to Love whatever it is that we Hate – to embrace everything with Love and Acceptance – to go towards all our fears and sadness with love, kindness and compassion... The story goes that we have both wolves in us – and the question is which one do we listen to? And the answer is that it is the one we feed – the one that we give most attention to.

I could hear the Wolf of Hate constantly reminding me of what I had lost, how awful things were and how they could get worse – I was a nuisance, people would be fed up with me etc... on and on it would go – there are disasters round the corner – isolate yourself, you are washed up now – be ashamed... The Wolf of Hate invited me to continue to think like this – to feed it... and also there was the voice of the Wolf of Love – you're OK, you have done so well, you have a wonderful family and friends who you love and who love you – this is an exciting time – how can you use all these experiences to help yourself and others in the world... Be kind to yourself, allow yourself to ask for and receive help – stay connected to others... and I could choose to feed this wolf with more love and compassion....

I was in the Caravan – among trees and with few other people around, empty Caravans standing in rows. The mountains rising up around me. It was evening, a full moon and few stars... I took my little dog – my own tame Wolf, and wrapped up against the chill of the evening, we went out for a walk. I could feel the fear clutching at me – as my mind was tempted to go into imagining horrors out there – the horrors of the dark – and I think it was again my Mindfulness Practice which supported me through this time – because as I walked I did a Walking Meditation Practice – I deliberately Noticed the contact of my feet with the ground on each Step.
I counted them, Step One, Step Two,
And I breathed into each step,
Breathing In, Breathing Out
Bringing the attention into just this moment,
Letting go of all the thoughts.
And just being in this moment.

And I came back to the warmth of the Caravan, made a cup of Hot Chocolate – comfort food – and sat with Toby. I saw so clearly how I had been listening to the Wolf of Hate on and off since the Haemorrhages – and for a moment I wanted to get rid of him – let him go – and then I thought no, I need to keep both Wolves. Both have things to tell me – and I need to love them both. I sat down and painted a picture – to remind myself that when the wolves came visiting, to just accept them both… I did not have to listen to them, but I could hear them with compassion.

I slept then – without fear, warm in my caravan – at peace somehow.

The next day Toby and I continued our walk further into the woods. The wolves were still there but I was no longer frightening myself with them. But as I walk further, the trees get darker and closer. I can't see my way, I felt nervous of stumbling and getting lost. Thoughts of being here alone in the dark. And I remember the wolves, just there, out of sight and I realised I was scaring myself. And I smiled and took a breath, walked slowly, just feeling each step, just present in this moment.

As I walked, I noticed in the distance the sound of running water and I followed the sound and it got louder and then suddenly I saw a stream tumbling its way through the woods. I decided to follow the stream. After a while, the trees thinned out and light was coming in through the branches. I saw beside me the path that I had lost some time ago. And stepping out now on to the path, I saw a gate. I walked up to the gate and opened it and knew that I had come to the end of the woods.

Chapter 19: Out of the Woods and Building a Camp

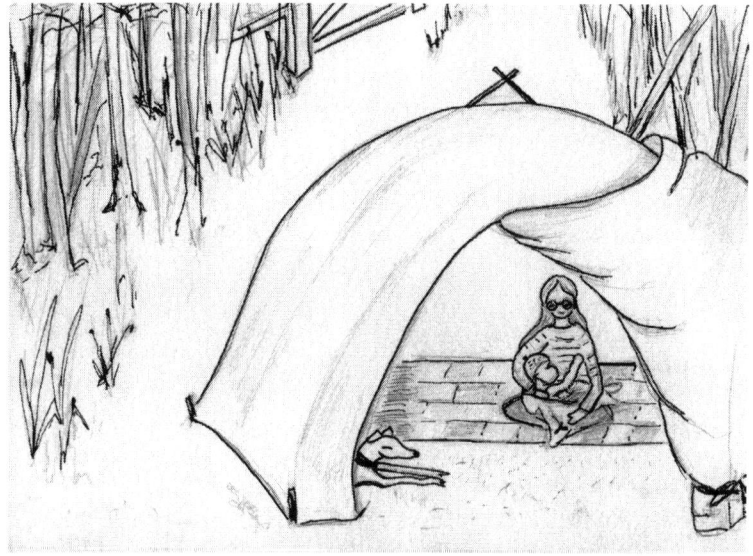

As I step through the gate and out of the woods, I seem to see a great empty plain in front and around me. Behind me are the woods. And I decide to stay just there, near to the woods and the stream, and build a camp. I didn't know it then, but I was to stay there for the next five years, journeying to and fro across the plain. I suppose I was on a discovery of this new life – this new person that I had become, my little dog at my heels. Visited by my family, going out to work driving my lovely red Beetle.

'Where am I now?', I ask myself. 'How is my head?' What is happening in my brain now? Where is the mud of the Tsunami?

Most of the mud has gone from my brain, so I can see the landscape of the brain now as if I were standing on top of a building or a high hill. Some places are clear, resting in pools of sunlight, and others are shrouded in mist. The ground is clear in some places, and in others the scarring from the mud is obvious. There are areas of the Tsunami-drenched brain where destroyed bits of memory and brain lie like rubble. In other places it is clear. I can see it as if in the distance.

But this is my mind now. It is what I live in and where I live. The ground is now clear enough to walk on. I can walk here and begin to find my way around. It seems big, empty, and a little scary and then it is that I turn to my Mindfulness Practice and my image of the Cup – the sense of containment that it brings. With this new awareness comes such a strong and overwhelming sensation of fatigue. Everything I do seems to be exhausting. Nothing seems simple – I spend a lot of time trying to work out and understand what is going on – that automatic knowing of the familiar has not returned. Each task is as if for the first time.

I turn to poetry and to the rhythm of poems. The simplicity of the words soothe me. I can understand them as I cannot understand long explanations.

I carry on with my everyday life, the daily tasks familiar – yet still for me now they are always done with new eyes. There is exhaustion in that. I discovered that automatic pilot – not having to think too much about everyday familiar tasks – is restful – I miss it now – everything seems to require such an effort of attention and memory.

BUT gradually I learn again – what I have known before and then forgotten – to be just in this moment. It is when I look at the whole view – the whole journey – that things can seem too much. Go back to the lesson of first walking in that Tsunami mud, just this moment – and walk with curiosity, allowing new eyes, allowing to see, to just be, and trust. Here I am, with my Camp just behind me, the woods and all my knowledge and past life and friends... they are all still there, just now, here right now. Can I have the courage to keep opening to, and finding the joy in, this new landscape, these new eyes?

And this too I must, and will, get used to. The brain after all is just an organ of the body, and in the same way as a badly injured leg will no longer jump and climb as it once did, so the brain too has its new patterns and strengths and weakness.

Again my Mindfulness is so helpful because I can easily feel sorry for myself or begin one of those tiring and dispiriting thought cycles of 'isn't it awful about... that I can't... etc.' And I know I have a choice of where to go, where my mind goes, what type of thoughts I choose to stay with and encourage.

Walking out this morning on my way down to the shops, my mind churning around and searching, as minds do, for all the things that were wrong, for what I didn't like, and wanted to be different – I suddenly stopped. 'Why am I giving myself all this suffering?' I thought – and laughed too, because I just thought, already my path is covered with boulders and stones that creep into my shoes – obstacles I once would have managed, I can now go around.

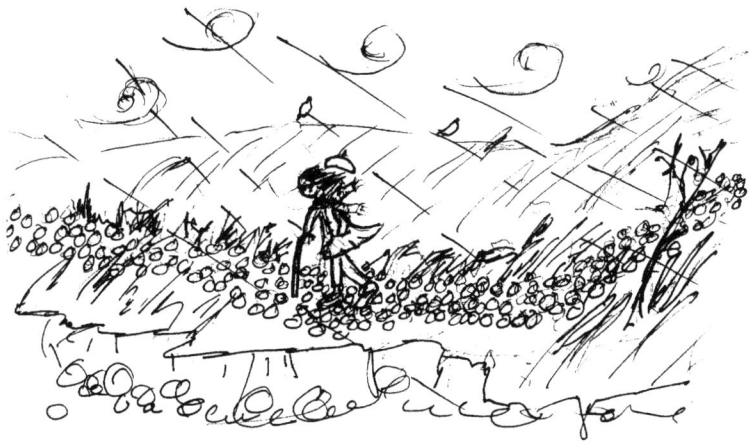

I seemed to live in two worlds. Out at work I was Training. I see looking back at my Journals that with my colleagues from the Centre for Mindfulness in Bangor, I taught a lot of residential Mindfulness Courses, training new teachers and running a Meditation Retreat. I worked from home as a Supervisor of Mindfulness Teachers and also using a Mindfulness led approach to therapy.

Supported by so many people. My dear colleagues were extraordinary in their kindness and patience. I was able to teach – to lead Meditation Practices, all that seemed intact. I could interact with others, hold the group. Where the brain injury showed up was in the in-between places – such as the times between the formal group training sessions. Again, colleagues quickly got used to this and in a way became my inner clock, because I didn't seem to have one now.

I could keep to the planned time of the training sessions – but once out and about, meal times, between sessions, I seemed to be unaware of time passing. So my colleagues would develop a way of herding me back – letting me know when and where I needed to be.

Because of the nature of our work, practising Mindfully, being aware of how we were moment by moment, with compassion and curiosity, we all seemed to manage this process – as did my students. The fact that I was able to teach, to remember the meditations and the theory, to engage in group and individual discussion, showed that I could still teach effectively. Yet in between, going to meals on time, organising the in-between time – I lost the time. It was as if I needed that quite rigid structure that there is in a training course. You do this now – and this now. Time is organised.

This has continued, years later now at home, retired, only my time to manage. I move constantly between knowledge and awareness of time passing. Just now, I realise, is a good example. It is dark outside – the village is asleep – it is 3.30am and I have started my day as I often do, with an awareness of NOW – what is here, around me, in my experience of me… now. I like the quietness, nothing much is moving – later the birds will start the day and the noise of the world around begins. My time world often seems a little apart from the rest of the world.

I think this is a part of the nature of Brain Injury. It is very pleasant in a way and only a problem when my inner time clock clashes with the timing and expectations of the outside world.

So Toby and I settle into our Camp. It is a strange experience, this sense of Camp on the edge of a plain, while I sit and look out of my bedroom window at the sea – that wonderful seascape that I have watched change, the weather go across, the birds flying, since the Tsunami. I drive out to work, and life goes on. I simply have these NEW EYES – the world is different. Maybe that was why I liked this idea of a Camp: it felt safe and apart from the everyday world and I needed that retreat in order to manage the noise, the movement – how quickly cars and people and situations and events change. There is endless movement and noise everywhere. Going into those always brilliantly and blindingly light Shops – constant movement and noise of the world – everyday life. Stepping out of my house and going anywhere busy was an assault – of noise, lights, doorways and passages.

But I learnt to manage this – and I think I stayed in my sense of the containment of the camp for the next five years because it gave me a sense of a refuge from the noise and din around me. To start with, inside my head, there was often so much movement, as if my brain itself was falling – flashing lights at the corner of my vision, the bombardment of noise. Sometimes my brain seemed quite blank – it would take me time to somehow reconnect with some coherent pattern of thought. At other times there was a confusing babble of thoughts and confusion.

I learnt to be with that, whatever my experience in my mind or body might be, by having that attitude which came from my Mindfulness Meditation Practice… kindness, patience, curiosity. Just sitting in THIS MOMENT – THIS MOMENT – THIS MOMENT – BREATHING. Several times a day I would go and 'sit on my cushion' – my meditation cushion or stool. Taking time, perhaps only five minutes or maybe 30 or 40 minutes of Sitting. And frequently just Noticing when things became too loud around me, the brain too confused, and I would simply:

STOP – whatever I was doing, wherever I was – either just stand still, or go and sit somewhere, anywhere – in the midst of something – on a bench in a Railway Station, into a Café for a Meditation Space.

SIT – and bring my attention to asking myself WHAT IS HAPPENING NOW? Just NOTICING – what is there in my body – sensations – in my mind – thoughts coming and going.

– BREATHING – following my in breath and out breath – this breath, this breath, this breath.

– LETTING GO of whatever is here and just simply following my breath – and GROUNDING – that sense of the body solid, here, on my seat.

And this might be a brief, 3–5 minute practice – even just a few moments – or I may sit for longer, depending on time and circumstances.
The longer practices were very steadying, allowing my often jumbled mind to settle. Or they just allowed me to PAUSE in the rushing chaos of the world – one deep CONSCIOUS BREATH could bring me back into a calm awareness of myself and my environment.

Sometimes it was good to do what we call a FORMAL PRACTICE – so I might take up to 45 minutes and sit down on a Meditation Cushion or Stool – But it was the frequent PAUSES – for a few moments or minutes, to become aware of how I was RIGHT NOW – with COMPASSION and KINDNESS towards whatever was going on for me – and it was, and is, a respite... these Pauses to gather – to turn towards ourselves with Kindness.

STOP... SIT... BREATHE

So this Mindfulness Practice was always there with me, sitting in my CAMP and out and about in the world.

I felt very joyous. So much had happened... the Weddings... and already my little granddaughter is running around... and now my Grandson N is born and later I begin to visit regularly to look after him when my daughter was at work.

We had such fun – I would load up the pushchair and we would go on adventures with Toby trotting along beside us. We walked along the path by the canal, fed the ducks, visited the ponies, played games, read books, watched television cartoons and his favourite programme, *Room on the Broom*. So many stories to be read.

And then something changes for me. Setting out towards the station to go home one day, I was walking along the towpath by the canal and I began to feel odd. A strange yet familiar sensation in my head, pain, a sense of falling. And then I found myself lying on the ground beside the canal, struggling to sit up. No one was around. It was early evening. I recovered quite quickly and, using my stick, walked into town to a nearby café and sat there with a coffee while I recovered. And then I carried on to the station and came home. I wasn't sure what had happened but later it became obvious I'd had a stroke and really it wasn't safe for me to be looking after the children anymore. And it was time for N to go to a lovely childminder and be playing with other children.

I started on a series of hospital appointments and investigations, up and down to Walton again for scans. There was always a chance of another haemorrhage or of some leaking from the site of the original aneurysm. But I did not want more surgery. There were risks both ways. But now in my 70s, I love being old and I decided to continue on as the risks of surgery seemed too great. I would trust and live whatever time I had. As I am writing this book, it is four years later and I'm still here. I'm glad I made that decision. Because my eldest daughter had lived with her brain injury since she was a baby, 40 years ago, this was not new territory to me or to my family.

I seemed to move between worlds. Sometimes in that nearby town with my daughter and her husband and now little N. Sometimes here in the village I live in with my son and family and little granddaughter. My dear step-grandson too, now looking at Universities. The years were rolling by.

I now have three young grandchildren and I can see the changes around me, my village, the world, the people I love. I saw a drawing I had done some time ago of a Buddha just sitting and beside it I had written:

Whatever comes, Let it come.
Whatever stays, Let it stay.
Whatever goes, Let it go

This is how I will live with the changes from my brain injury, the strokes.

I can see and feel the losses around me... and also feel the joy of just this moment... that wisdom of allowing whatever is, to be here.

I wrote a poem dated 8 March 2013.
But I did die.
Do they not know
They have a ghost
Walking among them?

And I drew my familiar picture that has become The Map, of the Rope Bridge... the wilderness then the mountain range. The Lightning strike and

Chapter 19: Out of the Woods and Building a Camp

the Forest... and now the Camp looking out over the great Plains... criss-crossed with paths... some dead ends, somewhere a maze... and I realised that this was the confusion... I was in a Maze... the maze of my new brain and I was walking the twists and turns of the maze... unable to see the past or future... just this place here now...

My Brain felt in another place... and suddenly it was as if I fell... reminding me of Alice in Wonderland and how she fell down the great tunnel inside the Rabbit Hole and, arriving at the bottom, I knew the place for the very first time.

I realised again, in a new way, that there was no turning back. 'Whatever comes... let it come.' And so I carry on... living my life in the Real world... but I think I found the Real world too noisy, too confusing, endless movement too fast for me... and so I lived my parallel life on the Plain, in the safe haven of my Camp.... every day a completely new adventure. Everything was new... I had new eyes.

After a while it was as if my CAMP became even more protected and separate to the noise and din and speed of the life out there in the world. I would come back to my camp now to gather strength and rest before I went back out to operate in the noisy, frantic and fast world.

Looking back as I write now, I think the safety of this sense of being in a Camp was because actually out there in the real world everything was just too big and loud... so loud. Everything... sound, sights, senses were shouted. And I found a way to stand slightly aside, so that the noise became indistinct.

And my face had changed again... as I write, a little voice in my head says, 'oh no, not your face again... everyone will think you spend your life looking in the mirror'! I smile, and I do... whenever I go into the bathroom I look in the mirror... why? It is somehow to reassure myself that I am here... I did not die. But then of course I notice that I do not... to me anyway... look the same... and there is always a shock from that, like being knocked off course... how can this be... and then that curiosity, 'well, who are you then?'

And I remind myself of my Acceptance meditation practice...
'Stop... Pause... Breath... Feel your feet on the FLOOR...
Turn Towards
Open your arms to whatever is here.
Just be here
Stay open to whatever comes
Say "I am fine just the way I am"
Whatever comes... let it come
Whatever goes let it go.
Breathing...'

End of All Things

Here now
At what seems like the end of all things,
I feel the stir and movement of my breath
As though great wings of angels are near,
Calling me to let go,
To allow myself to trust
Pausing where the light changes
To rest in the cracks between light and dark
Where day and night merge.
The place where peace and fear meet
Where all things – like the breath
Turn and turn again.
(Jody Mardula)

Chapter 20: Paths that Open and Close

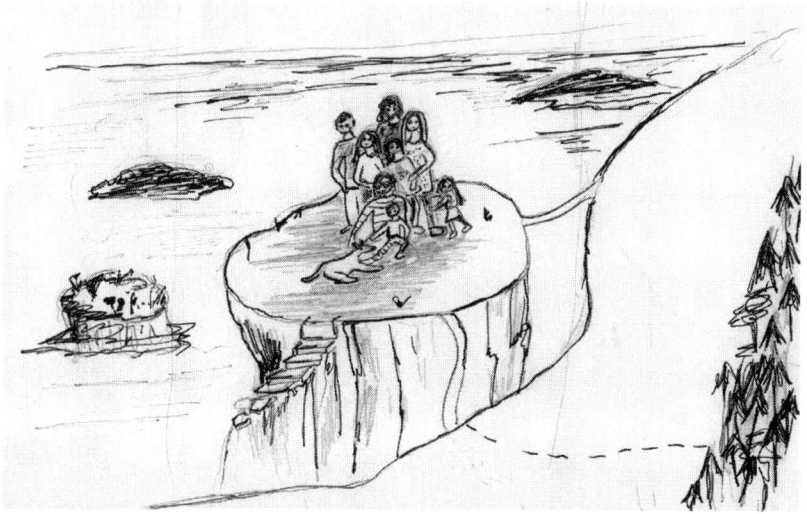

After being in the Camp for a while, I begin to experience the sense of us all living on different islands. I was not wanting anything to be different – but just acknowledging it is how it is. There is a sadness in that – but I think it is the final acceptance of the change the Brain Injuries made in me and therefore in everyone in my family. You can never go back – there is always joy and sadness. There is great joy in being a Grandmother – and also that sadness that I wasn't the Grandmother I would have been – but this is just life – with or without brain injury, we change. Things are rarely as we expect. Perhaps there is more finality – or obviousness about the changes that come from traumas and injuries.

When I go into a place of anger and regret – which I sometimes do – and rail against it – this is not helpful. A while ago, I was watching the Invictus Games – thinking of the madness of what we do to each other as humans. War injuries that have changed people's lives. So many have completely devastating physical injuries and yet people find their way through. Of course, we do not see the mental anguish. The dynamics which I talk about here – the impact on others of our injuries. How it can build on or destroy what was there before. There is no better or worse here – just how it is.

So what have been the losses? Well the relationship I might have had with my Grandchildren... but that is fantasy – I am what I am to them and we have a wonderful relationship. They did not know me any other way. The loss of my status – and I have come to smile at that. As is often the case, I had not realised how much I had enjoyed my work and being in a role where I had authority – where I could develop and make things happen – and feel worthwhile and sometimes important!

My Brain Haemorrhages brought both gains and losses.

The gains have been that slowing down – forced to Pause – to Stay More Still – and in that to SEE more clearly – those hours early on when I could only sit in bed and watch the sky and sea change out beyond my window.

And that has carried me through – became HOW I managed – how I learnt to ACCEPT and not fight against what was happening, the losses and the changes.

The walks I go on – to the beach – finding somewhere flat for walking – my little wooded park – nearby.

How I learned to really SEE the trees – the sky – to hear the birds – because my Mind – my head... is stilled. Before I would often go for much longer walks – but during the walk I would be thinking and planning. I might be organised – with binoculars, note books, pens. Going somewhere – getting somewhere.

Or maybe as I walk I would be busy planning my life – dinner tonight – things needing to be DONE – paid – bought – organised, my next holiday. Solving a problem. All the daily chores of life and work would accompany me so often. Although, I would pause in my walks to Meditate... to breathe... to notice... see what was around me... feel the sense of air on my body... notice my thoughts, let the mind still... – but pretty soon, as I resumed the walk, my busy mind would start again.

Now my mind had changed – it was much quieter. That caused problems in terms of remembering things and getting things done – progressing, as it were, with life and work. My aim had been to keep this pace of life and use my Mindfulness Practice. Indeed, it had been woven into my life before the Brain Injury. There was great loss – and also this calm, still spacious mind. I was to find so much more compassion – it seemed to have emerged from the ruin and the blood.

And I do miss going for those long walks from before the bleeds – up hills, over mountains, wonderful views. Now my mind is slow to plan – I do not have the physical stamina to go so far or fast... I cannot drive to the places of beauty

I used to visit – too inaccessible – too far. I find, so unlike me, that I like to drive, even walk, in familiar places. I miss the mountains – and I have lost what was an unthinking trust in my body's capabilities and stamina… the confidence in my ability to know where I was – how to get back – my sense of direction. At first that seemed quite gone – now – later – a little returned. But I have not got the stamina to take the risk of just going off somewhere – knowing that I do not have the capability to cope with any eventuality.

Now I knew I could easily tire, lose my balance and fall – forget where I was – how I got here and how to get back. Being out somewhere far from people – that old confidence that I would have had, had gone. These are the results of Brain Injury – the changes. If I had been younger I imagine I may have been able to develop more physical and mental stamina again. But more than the physical, I would need my Perception to sharpen – my Balance to adjust – the ability to recall direction – to build my brain and physical strength.

To some extent I did, but mostly I have built the emotional stamina to allow and accept my new limitations. To view them not so much as limitations but as gateways – to see things differently – different intentions for a walk. To find as much beauty wherever I was. The difference was in seeing and being with what was already here – what I found around me – than always going away to somewhere else to find it. Interesting. I knew this before. But somehow was caught up in this seeking outside.

So now – as the years pass by – I often do exactly the same every day – go on the same walk. Much slower, not for as long, not getting very far – and yet every day is different.

Sometimes I go somewhere with family or friends that brings great joy and pleasure. I notice that anything new also brings exhaustion. I may not have walked any further, but the brain is taking in new material – a new place – and that is very tiring. I think that is one of the things that I often feel is not understood – the huge impact of the environment on me since the Brain Injury – a short visit to somewhere NEW will result in exhaustion quite quickly.

This happened all the time at first, and then got a little better. But now, over the years I do know my limitations, and to some extent have accepted them. There is learning that comes from that – the restrictions to short walks in safe nearby places. When I use the learning from my Meditation Practice – then there are no boundaries or restrictions to experience. There is awareness – just by stopping and looking at the sky – feeling the air on my face – hearing the birds. This has as much wonder as any other experience. My less busy mind is also a more aware, more spacious and more knowing mind.

The walk I went on today is the same as yesterday's – but what I noticed, how it felt, the sounds, the weather, the shape of the sky and the movement of the trees – they were all unique to today.

> ### Neuro Notes 5: Acceptance
>
> Learning to accept stroke and brain injury problems, rather than struggle against them, is often an enormous challenge. It is normal to want to turn back the clock, and for everything to be the way it was before. It is entirely natural to want to 'beat' the injury by trying to carry on as before.
>
> Jody had cultivated a mindful acceptance of difficulties over many years, but even so, did not always feel accepting of or curious about her difficulties, especially after the second stroke. Like many people with a stroke, Jody had to learn to live with exhaustion and pain, slipping memories and a crashing brain, and with new emotions and relationship changes.
>
> Jody found that reconnecting with her mindfulness practice and focusing on the present moment helped her to be more accepting of the way things were. Being in the 'here and now', rather than worrying about the future or feeling regret, tends to make our difficulties more bearable.
>
> Talking with people in similar circumstances, or finding new and meaningful activities and relationships after the stroke or brain injury can make acceptance easier. People can find positives in the changes – for example, Jody valued her new, slower pace of life, and her quieter and more spacious mind.
>
> For some people, family relationships and friendships become more important. There may be new opportunities in life, as well as difficulties.
>
> Some people find it hard to accept their stroke or brain injury and its effects. As a result, they may be reluctant to take part in rehabilitation or to work towards improvement.
>
> Working towards improvement is a sign that the person can acknowledge their situation, and that they want to make the best of it. This can take a lot of courage, and the person may need reassurance and support in order to keep going.
>
> Learning to accept and to live with the effects of a stroke or brain injury can take months or years. Patience is essential; acceptance cannot be forced, only encouraged. The person and their family may need to grieve for things that have been lost, as they learn to adjust to a new direction in life.

Part 6: In the Camp

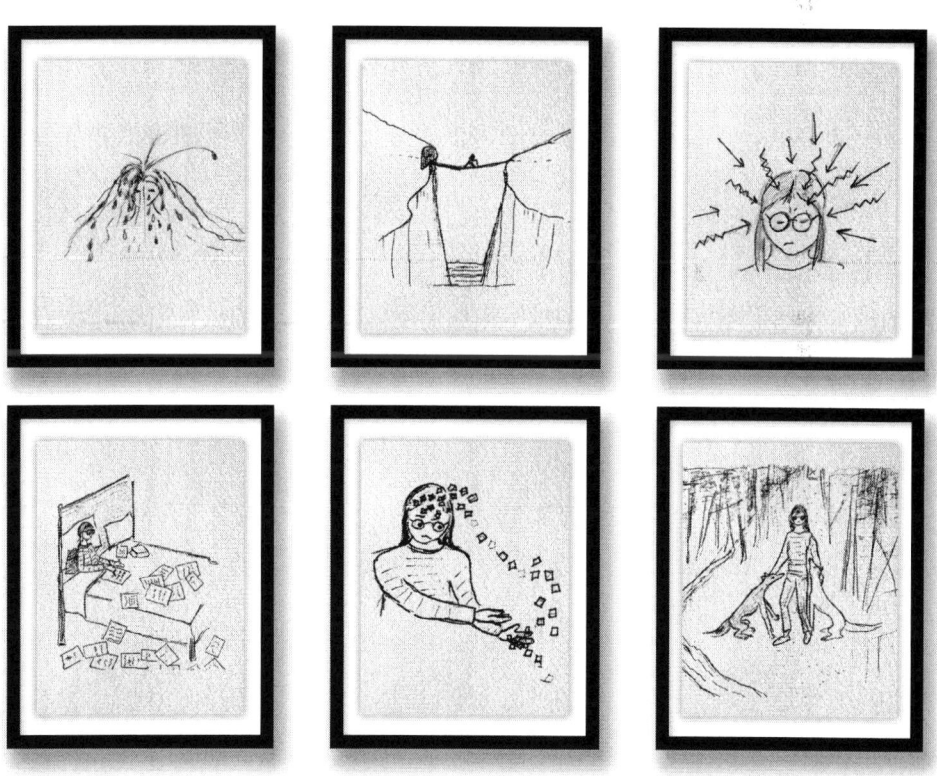

Chapter 21: Falling Mind

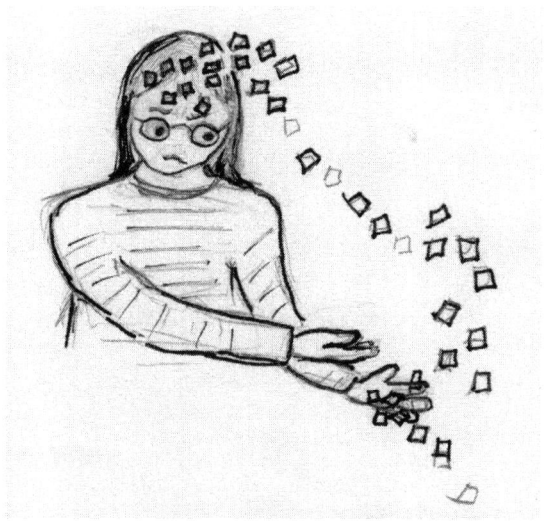

It can be hard to really capture what it is like to continually forget and reorganise material in the memory without any sense of control.

I often almost physically feel the information as a sensation. It is as if the memory slips or falls away in chunks. I grasp at it as it goes, but once it starts to slip, I may capture and retain some part of it – but mostly it is just gone. If at least I am aware it was there and is gone, I have more chance of retrieving some of it. If I try to grab it, it is more likely to go.

Slipping memory affects every part of my life. We revolve around memory – of tasks, what is done, what to do, who did what, who we are, what we like, what we don't like. There are many ways in which memory goes – and I can hear you say 'we all do this' – and indeed we do. Often it can happen when we are tired, overloaded, unwell, or at certain stages of life – menstrual and menopausal – and as a part of the aging process. But there is a different quality and absoluteness to the post-brain injury memory loss that I experience.

This morning I suddenly had one of those welcome moments when I could clearly see what I wanted to write today. I would write about the next stage of my journey – memories of times and events were coming to mind. I made myself comfortable and picked up my pad of paper and pencil and as I did that and turned to look again at what I had been thinking about saying. Then I had one of those moments – we will all know them – when I couldn't quite remember. What was it I was going to write? But Brain Injury memory loss has a different quality to my previous memory losses and confusions. There is an absoluteness to it.

This morning, as I notice this happening, I am determined to follow the thread of awareness and I stand here with a large pad of paper and pencil to write down the process as it falls around me. Once I have something written down, I know I have more chance of reclaiming at least some of it… and I want to record it for this book.

So often I forget I saw something or said something – it tumbles away and often I know it – see and feel it go. I go cold, like now. I want to get it, catch it whatever it is; sometimes I can – often I cannot.

I feel fear. There is a strong sense of being out of control – that it is important not to forget this… This process has been with me since I first had the Brain Haemorrhage. Sometimes it is stronger than at other times – certainly how tired I am, and if I am in an unfamiliar environment or distressed, affects it. But always, always things are slipping. Sometimes it seems as if they tumble away, sometimes they float away.

And then I forget I even saw and thought something, until suddenly I see it again – know I knew this before – try to grasp it – and sometimes I do – but it has taken years to learn to do even that. The reason is that my brain does not easily organise material – so even when I remember, that memory has to go somewhere, be stored – it is almost as if I am in an office with piles of papers but nowhere to put them.

But yes, sometimes I do see it – and I do have a system – and sometimes I remember what it is and on those days I will see clearly, as I do now, what is happening. I will manage to catch and record some of my thoughts – even write them down – which can be good because it is more concrete. But then I have to both remember that I wrote it down and also where I put it. Just going out of the room – or taking a phone call – and all that can go. Maybe I don't remember where I put it or even that it happened.

So that process, 'I am sure I wrote that down', 'where did I put it' – I hear the 'we all do this' going on – perhaps – but not to the degree that happens with Brain Injury.

When I capture and write something down, it has to be put somewhere. Maybe it is a note on a pad, a document in a file, a chapter for this book – but once it is out of sight I may never find it again. The chances are that even its existence will go – so I write another version – goodness knows how many times I have written different chapters about the same thing for this book!

I find that now, all these years on, I am better at this game with my mind. I know this, ah, I think, I can feel the slipping sensation, something is going – and maybe I can make a note that will help me to pick it up later. If I can, as I am doing now – just write down or type whatever is here – make it concrete – then that is good. I have a feeling that I am repeating myself here again – well, it all has to be organised into what is relevant for me and my life. Mostly we do this out of awareness. I think that I do this with lots of things or I would not manage life at all. Communications – conversations with people – the organisation of memory and plans – or what I have done – or what I was going to do or say – that is very prone to just fall away.

I wonder if I am communicating the utter despair – the almost sick feeling as I see it go. It is like standing in a shower of hard pieces of something – hitting me as they fall. Or it is as if I am being mentally sick with everything inside me being expelled from my body.

Today, at this moment, I see so clearly how the twin experiences of forgetting and not being able to organise things have had such a great influence on how I manage life and work, post-haemorrhages. Everything is made much harder and more of a struggle. It is so much more tiring – and then that feeds into the whole thing.

Right now, as I write this, I am trying to capture it. I am writing this chapter because I had one of those sudden moments of seeing clearly what I do. I think it has been, and is, one of the more distressing ongoing aspects of having a brain injury.

Whatever I do, it gets worse. I may continue to retrieve bits of memory for a while – but anything can go at any moment. It may go for a while or it may go, it seems, forever.

Or it may come back, but scrambled – words mixed up – and this then affects what I can remember and what I can communicate. My actions day to day depend on this – on what I remember and communicate to myself.

To others I know it can seem muddled – it is why I cannot teach any more. Why increasingly, although I KNOW what I am doing, and what ideas I have – I avoid meetings. Because as I talk – engage – become enthusiastic, have ideas, it will all begin to fall. So I start to stumble – and if I am alone – or with one or two close people who know me well, I can carry on. They will often then tell me back what I have lost, but you cannot be like that in everyday life. You just look muddled, stupid and of course, increasingly for me now, OLD.

This process of forgetting and the tumbling and scrabbling of memory, knowledge and experience contributes to the chaos that can accompany me through life now. I might be on a journey – out shopping – cooking – doing pretty well anything. I never know where I may suddenly forget – perhaps what I am doing or where I am going and how to get there.

I will notice that what I thought and am doing is beginning to go. I try so hard to put attention on it, stay with it, not let it fall...

Right now, as I am writing, it is early in the day. Light is just creeping over the window. I am sitting here on my bed – scribbling – trying to capture what I just saw so clearly about the slipping and falling mind. I had to get it down Now Now, before it is too late.

But actually I can feel the void right now – it has taken a lot of energy to write just this probably rather muddled bit. I know I have to stop now. I will go down and make a cup of green tea and take some paracetamol for the headache that this concentration has brought on. I will breathe, and sit, and maybe read a poem or two, until I can return to this theme. I do not want to let it go now. It is such an important part of this journey – of the understanding of people with Brain Injury about how the memory is affected, as presumably it must so often be. It is so important to this book.

I want people to understand that yes, all the props, the things they so often suggest – make a list, have a notebook, talk into your phone and leave a message for yourself... yes – I do all of that – AND... AND... you also have to then remember that you did that – where you put it etc... There can be a place of utter blankness where there are very few threads to grasp at – and then the inability of putting them anywhere at all – so of course they too fall away. And the unpleasant sensation – a near parallel to being sick or fainting – that can accompany it.

I go down now for my tea. I am putting this notebook on my pillow and I will leave some post its on the stairs to remind me that this is what I am doing – to come back to it when I have drunk the tea. I have a note here that my granddaughter, who is now six and who I was with yesterday, wrote for me to take with me when I went home (just down the road). It tells me what she wanted me to bring back for her... 'Grandma – I want you to bring "Grandma Biscuits" and toys like pepper pig toy'. I smiled, and kept this note. I think she knows already that I need reminders. And it was so useful because I did bring them back as she asked. I love that totally non-judgemental acceptance that children have – and the practicality of it. She was making sure I didn't forget what she wanted – and also she was helping me.

The chances were that I could have totally forgotten what she wanted in the process of making the tea, if I didn't have the note.

… So I am back now from my trip for Green Tea. I am planning now – I need to type this up on my PC – and then save it in the right place – and then print it. I have to have everything I write printed out or I am likely to completely forget what I wrote. There is something more concrete about sheets of words on paper that I can hold, compared to words on a screen that I may never find again! This too requires memory. I have to remember that I wrote this. (There are endless notebooks and notes around this house where I have written a chapter and then forgotten. I come across them from time to time, like notebooks of ghosts from my past.) Then I have to be organised to type it all up and FILE IT IN THE RIGHT PLACE ON THE COMPUTER (ditto above – there are endless files scattered around different places on the PC).

Have I communicated this, I wonder? It is easy to say – 'we all do this' – or 'it happens because you are older'. It is the dual process of memory slipping and the reduced capacity to organise material that makes it all so absolute. But this Brain Injury memory loss and slipping is NOT what the memory losses that we all have were like before my Haemorrhages.

That is why for me, Mindfulness has been such a gift. Because the experience of forgetting, the muddled sick feeling of trying to make the brain organise things – just like constantly putting paper into a nice neat pile, only for it to fall in a heap on the floor, perhaps being swept up. Everything falling away, and the utter despair that can bring – no no – racing about – don't go, I need this, I need to know where I am going, what I am doing, no no, I want to remember that wonderful moment… catch it… catch it… as it slips away.

But there are moments when I NOTICE this is happening – it isn't always there, sometimes and some things get remembered, can be recalled particularly with the right cues – but there are the times of slipping – and then I can turn to my Mindfulness practice and tell myself to:

STOP – to PAUSE.
TO Notice my BREATH.
To become aware of the contact of my body, whether it is my feet on the floor – standing – or feet on floor and body on chair – SITTING or whole body LYING DOWN…
STOP and just notice my BREATHING.
This breath IN and this breath OUT.
Breathing In and Breathing out.

For those moments there is nothing to do but meditate – so simple – nothing else needs to be thought about or done – just feel the body standing or sitting and notice and follow the in breath and out breath. TAKING A BREATHING SPACE. And that allows an acceptance – allowing things to be just as they are, trusting myself to find a way but to know that just now I need to let go, and settle myself into calm. Not in any way trying to remember or capture what is lost... Let it go... smile... breathe.

I find after that I am then much calmer, not so caught up in trying to remember to grasp whatever is gone or going. And somehow there is something that is KIND about the breath, about giving ourselves to those moments where we are not striving and trying to do something or get somewhere – but just allowing ourselves to be as we are, in this moment, breathing, supported by whatever we are standing or sitting on.

And then I can say to myself, 'Let it go', whatever it is I was trying to grasp – and ironically, often once I am relaxed and calm, some of it may come back.

Later my memory changes again – there is a different quality to it – this earlier post-haemorrhage memory seems pretty good in comparison.

No Ticket to Return
Great slabs of memory
Tumble from my brain,
Sometimes I feel them as they fall
'Oh' – there one goes again.

There even is a place nearby
Where they can all remain
A lost property for memories
But no ticket to reclaim.

And there's another type of loss
That others see – not me
That were not even labelled lost
Now no-one's property

Perhaps all of me – my brain will go
Into that no man's land,
My ticket now that's lost and gone
Just left with knowing 'something's wrong'
(Jody Mardula)

Chapter 22: Perception

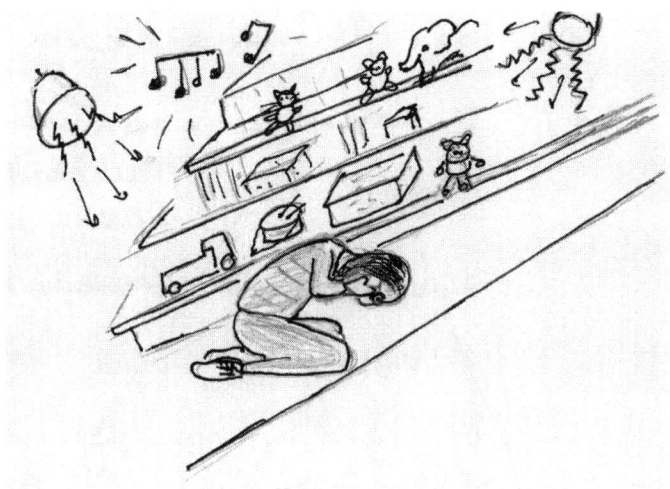

A stranger in the midst of strangers

The more I went out and began to try and pick up the threads of my life, the more I began to realise that the effects of the Brain Haemorrhage were not going to go away – or even 'get better'. Perhaps I just needed to continue to find new ways to be in this changed mind – this changed world.

As I began to fully experience the day-by-day changes, it was as if I was a toddler – exploring a new and often bewildering world – seeing things for the first time, finding ways in which I have to adapt.

Faces and places

I simply no longer seemed to recognise faces… other than people I saw regularly, I tended not to recognise people I met in the street. For the first time since the Brain Injury, this led to me seeming to ignore people… They would speak to me and I didn't have a clue who they were. I would know I had said something 'wrong' – like 'I don't know who you are' – by the look on their face.

Yet at the same time, I didn't recognise people as 'strangers' and so I would talk to people I didn't actually know as if we were old friends… There was a gain from this. I met some wonderful people who I would never otherwise have known. I also had a strange sense of belonging in a community… there was no separation. And those people would accept me just as I was – they had nothing to compare me to.

But it was not always comfortable with people I did know. I often didn't recognise them until they spoke, and even then not until I had some clue to fit them into place... and it was disturbing because as I realised who someone was – longtime friend or even family – they still looked different, so in a way it wasn't them. Eventually I adjusted to that and learned not to tell people I didn't recognise them, because it was upsetting for them. I learned a new level of sensitivity.

In the same way, going to places... walking down familiar streets... they were no longer familiar. I had to relearn them. Everything seemed to need to be re-seen – re-perceived and re-learnt. Eventually this too became a part of the New Normal. I adjusted. It is just how life is, only brought forward in time. It was a bit like anyone of us going back to somewhere we knew many, many years ago. It might not be quite as we remembered it. We see it with new eyes. As I recall this and write about how intense this was at the beginning of this journey, I feel that sadness, as we do when we go back to a place and find it much changed. Or when we re-meet an old friend and find that things are no longer the same between us. We all change. It was simply that I had changed too quickly – I was a time traveller.

Moving objects

I had not previously realised how much of our environment is moving. Interestingly, the movement of trees in the breeze – the clouds, the birds – did not have the same effect on me as man-made movement.

Just as I had experienced that sense of the road coming up to hit me and the tunnels closing in on that car journey home from the hospital – there were places and situations that had the same effect.

It was a couple of years before I could comfortably watch television – and even now I only watch a few programmes. There are many I will immediately turn off – anything with bright shooting colours – a lot of movement. In those early days I could not tolerate it at all. I was blinded by the light from the screen and anything moving quickly. I would feel sick – as though I might fall over. Moving colours and shapes that dart out of the screens at me like arrows – in a permanent 3D film experience. This bombardment from screens (loud noise was also intolerable) – just being out and about, there are so many screens in so many places. And they move. I am OK with information screens, if they move very, very slowly – but of course they don't. And if the screen (in a train station, for example) has too much information on it and keeps moving, I cannot look at it.

I became aware of how much of our lives are lived through screens. In many situations there are voice announcements – but often they are too quick for me. I was living on a slower planet than everyone else. Later, of course, I had to learn to manage computer and phone screens. With my own I can have them adapted – low light – movement at a pace that I can manage – but I can't adjust the outside world. So I had to adjust my inside world.

That is what we mean by recovery, only it is not so much recovery as relocation to a new person and world.

Shopping environments

Going into any building – whether shop or restaurant or public place – can bring new obstacles. I am immediately aware of the sense of the space – whether it feels calm and spacious, in which case I can find my way around, stop and look at things, easily make decisions, find where to pay.

But many shops are rather like Amusement Arcades for me – and many are to some degree unbearable.

I could go into our local shops in the village easily because they are relatively quiet, and I can stay focused. It is hard enough to look at any shelf of goods and remember what I want and make a choice. I need a quiet, still environment in which to do that.

I have adapted by learning my way round nearby supermarkets that I choose to use. I know what to expect, and how to navigate them. Unfortunately they always change the layout of goods from time to time and that causes me difficulty and takes me time to relearn the route.

When I first went into my familiar local supermarket I was overwhelmed. The long aisles seemed too narrow and appeared to slope upwards – rather like the road in the tunnel had on my way back from hospital. If there was also loud music or announcements, I would have to go out. I wanted to hide from the brightness of the lights and the noise and all the colour on the shelves, which seemed to move in the corner of my eyes. All around me solid things seemed to move. There were people and trolleys – everything seemed... and still seems... huge, fast and noisy.

I learnt to visit one or two aisles – no more – on each visit. Luckily my local supermarket had fruit and veg, milk and dairy and some ready meals in those first two aisles, so I could manage by just going to them. Later, I learned how to do internet shopping again – difficult because this involved a screen and choices – but I could do it over a period of time – and once my family helped me to establish a list, I could just keep ordering that.

Over time I have learned how to manage – how to filter out the noise and light and movement, for the most part. However if I am tired – or too many things have changed and are not as expected – then I can still experience the whole thing crashing. My head simply stops working, I do not know what I am doing and simply have to get out of the store – or… if there is a café, go and sit there until my mind has readjusted.

We constantly move through so much noise – so much activity seems to be confined in noisy bright buildings with endless passages, rows of objects and the need to make choices. New stores – big stores with escalators – cafés and restaurants that so often have music – noise – distractions – It is so hard to find a peaceful, still building.

I will just mention our local – very big and no doubt excellent – super toy store – which even now I can hardly bear to be in. I need to know just what I want – where to find it – and get out quickly.

The first time I went in there for Christmas presents for my grandchildren I couldn't get out. I felt I was going to be sick – it was frightening. The high shelves of brightly coloured toys… the long narrow aisles to walk down, with the shelves seeming to lean forward and the boxes seeming to topple towards me. Bright blinding lights. Things bleeping and playing electronic tunes – a cacophony of noise overlaid by the insult of constant announcements… I had thought I would wander around looking at things and getting ideas. The first time I went in there, I simply got so overwhelmed and bewildered by it all, I just wanted to curl up on the floor. I froze – I couldn't think – I didn't know how to get out or what to do – and – as so often happens, because people are usually so kind – someone noticed and helped me to find my way out. I remember her making sure I knew where I was going – how to get home. People are so kind.

And now, much later, there are places I simply know to avoid – or to go with someone else who can help… or having the safety of knowing there is someone there who understands… who will just say 'tell me what you want and I will take you to it'.

I am a woman who has travelled the world – often alone – travelled on long train journeys as a young child – I could find my way around anywhere. But I can no longer find my way around the changed landscape of my mind.

I am writing about this because I find it very hard to communicate to other people just how the world can be for me.

I think there are probably several things that go on here. It is very hard for us to accept unwanted change in other people and perhaps particularly in those we love. We want them to be well – we don't want them to suffer – we want to have hope for them – we want them to be the same as they were.

There are particular difficulties, I think, that come with Brain Injury because it is unseen – the wound to the brain is invisible – our love wants them to recover. But it is simply harder to see… we can see the changes and scars of physical damage – in a way that we cannot see the scars of brain damage. Perhaps the only measuring rod you have is how much like the person they were before. That is what people so often mean by Recovery – be as you were before.

But of course, just like a badly broken limb may leave us with a limp, or an amputation leads to needing so much adjustment, others have to come to terms with that change in the injured person. All illnesses – maybe life threatening, like the changes from cancers and so many other ills of the body – all illness and injuries can change how we are – how we see and respond to life. Emotional damage and trauma impacts greatly on how we see ourselves, the person we are. And so can a damaged brain leave us with bits lost, rearranged, different. It is so hard for everyone concerned.

I understand that… I have been through several stages of how to come to terms with my changed world. How I have recovered memories and learning and skills, learnt to adapt and do things differently. I have had to learn to like myself again – to accept myself as I am with all the bits (as ever) I would like to be different – and to know that when anyone discounts me, 'oh we all do that', 'oh it's just like…', I think 'NO IT'S NOT'. This comes from an accelerated need to accept changes that might have taken a lifetime to emerge – and to learn to go towards being with things as they are now and not searching for how they were then. Loss and grief – but also out of the ashes something NEW grows. Not 'the same' – but different… even if unseen.

Chapter 23: The Trouble with Travelling

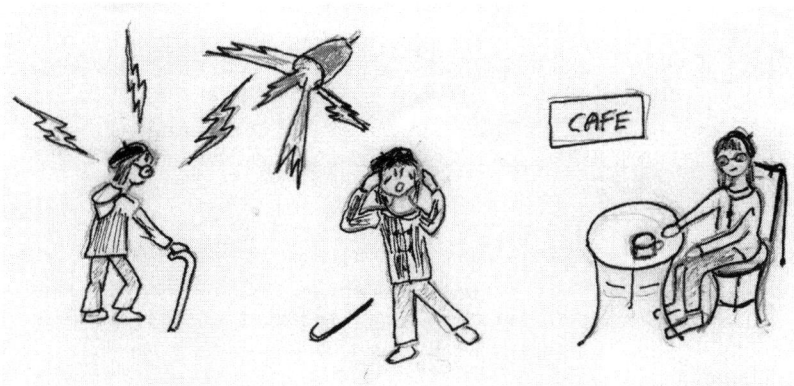

I just had a disaster with typing this chapter. Just as I had nearly finished it I pressed something that managed to accidently delete it all. Groan. Irretrievable.

And in some ways that felt rather like many of the journeys I have made since the Haemorrhages. Accidental moves, not having planned for something, and suddenly everything can go to pieces.

These things of course happen in everyday life for all of us, but I have found I am far more accident prone, more likely to mess up something, be somewhere at the wrong time or wrong place. All those sorts of things that I would do occasionally before are now far more likely since my brain injuries.

So any journey now needs two things. Patience and kindness towards myself when I mess up rather than berating myself! Having to do things over and over again. And Preparation. Prepare in advance, get the information you need, write it down, have a survival package with you.

I have always travelled a lot, and enjoyed it and believed I could deal with anything. One of the great losses for me from the damage of my brain injury is that I cannot easily travel, could not fly, and would not be able to travel anywhere unfamiliar alone. I always used to pride myself on that. From first taking seven hour train journeys to my first Boarding School aged eight, a long time ago on Steam Trains where everything was slower – to travelling abroad, hitchhiking, relying on my wits – to now, when the simplest journey needs to be planned, written down, lists made, a 'survival' bag taken with me.

After my initial brain injury, the first journeys on public transport that I had to go on alone involved catching a bus to my nearest town and then travelling to Hospital outpatients.

For any journey, I need to plan in detail, including checking timings and time of day. I have little awareness of time or how long things are taking now. My old ability to have some idea of the time of day and what to do next seems to have gone. Early on I quite often arrived at my destination to find that all the shops, or wherever it was I wanted to go to, were shut or just shutting. So my planning started with post its everywhere to remind me to check the time.

I enjoyed travelling, and maybe much of that came from that lack of awareness of time, I think. My Brain damage seemed to have given me the ability to be just fully in this moment, not worrying about the past or what comes next. No hurry to be somewhere else. Ironically, that is one of the positive attributes we engage in Mindfulness Meditation. However, in everyday life, it does help to have a wider awareness!

My first journeys were on the Bus to Llandudno, which I knew very well. But on that occasion I did not write it all down. I remember the shock of that first journey because I did not recognise where we were – I had to ask the bus driver to tell me when to get off in the centre of town. This place that I knew so well I didn't recognise as I had before. I could have been arriving there for the first time. Once I got used to that, I enjoyed seeing things as if for the first time and gradually I realised that there was memory. I had a sense of my way around, where things were in some of the stores. There was a mix of familiarity and unfamiliarity. The other thing I had not bargained on, but also learnt to plan for, was that I tired so quickly, and when tired I would tend to forget what I was doing and why I was there and sometimes even how to get home.

When this happened I would usually go and sit down somewhere, ideally in a café, and just sit, rest. Then I would have to find the bus stop to go home. And sometimes this was not easy and again I came across the kindness of strangers – someone always helped me.

And the next time I went I did remember, but not entirely, not in the way I would have before. There always seemed, and often still seems, to be an element of doubt. So there is something about the recognising brain, previously taken for granted, no longer here. I have learnt to prepare as if for the first time – lists, notes, reminders, for every journey… for every eventuality.

But I learnt a useful lesson on that first adventure out. Wherever I was going, whether I knew it well or not, was best regarded as being visited for the first time, so not just assuming I knew where to go or where to get off.

So first on the list for planning going anywhere was a written plan, as if going for the first time.

I was also inclined not to remember how to get back, and as I did not hold times in my head, it was also good to write down all possible times, and the route back, what to do and who to contact if I was in need of help. This did matter, because there were times, particularly early on, when I would get very tired, everything would seem to crash, and it could be quite difficult and distressing to get back home. Years later, I still tend to do this. Sometimes I can get used to the way to go, and the layout of a building, only to find it has all been changed. You never know what is going to be thrown at you. And something like that, unexpected, can throw you completely because it is so exhausting having to adapt to it.

This was all good learning for when I first got the train up to my Hospital outpatients appointments in Liverpool, with a two-hour journey each way and at least four changes. I prepared as if for a day's outing, which in fact it was. Times of trains, details of where to change and how to spot the right station. Details of how to negotiate changing stations, some of which were quite complicated and involved two sets of escalators and going through two ticket checkpoints! Details of the later times in case I got lost along the way.

I remember the first time ending up on a bench, on the wrong platform, trying not to cry, clutching my bag, and having no idea where I was meant to be or where I had put my notes on the Stations. It was getting dark. What had happened, of course, was that I had overloaded my brain and crashed. I began to learn both to notice the signs of moving towards crashing, which meant having no idea where I was or what to do, and to be prepared for it.

This was where I first came across the kindness of people, as I was to so many times over the years. Someone would always come up to me, find out if I was OK, and often actually take me to where I needed to be. Again and again I came across this kindness from strangers. I learnt too to take a written sheet of where I was going that I could show to people. And contact numbers, always contact numbers – do not rely on remembering ANYTHING. EVER.

But gradually, with some crashes and disasters along the way, I learnt my way around again. I never remembered in the way I did before, but I developed a new way of reminding myself of information and remembering, soothing and coping.

And also, the constant need for checking. So I would prepare journeys – and any sort of event – first, and then take prompts with me, and also on my hand or in a notebook I would write what to do if I got lost, tired or upset or crashed. I was learning how to get together a Survival kit! – for Journeys, visits to Cinemas (although that is later and another story) and meeting people.

If anything went wrong or I got confused, upset or lost, I would stop. Take out whatever I needed to be comfortable for a while – my Kindle, my hot drink and biscuits – essential headache pills – and my shawl. Every survival pack needs a warm shawl – nothing for me is more comforting. I had also learnt to expect these events as normal parts of pretty much anything – a shopping trip – just out for a walk – always be prepared for a crash.

And years later this is still the same, although it happens far less frequently and less deeply, but still, if things are late, complicated, go wrong, I am quickly and easily exhausted by the brain activity that is needed to work things out. Of course, we would expect this from a physical injury – a badly broken leg may well tire quickly. People often talk of a physical injury that can still ache years later. I don't think for the most part we are so good at responding to the brain's needs. We can't SEE the brain. I wasn't so good, anyway. And all the very helpful friends and people around me usually went into giving me more information rather than, read your Kindle, wrap yourself up, eat chocolate and have a hot drink! Wherever you are. I have sat down on the Traffic Isle in the middle of a busy road, leaning against the railings to calm myself in this way before attempting to cross the next bit.

More information with Brain Injury may NOT be what is needed; indeed, it may be what pushes you over into a crash.

So the trouble with travelling is partly the need to be so prepared for every eventuality (and all that is in itself tiring – I can be exhausted with it all before I have even set out). It is so important to take your time with a brain injury.

If you need to miss a train, miss it. Ask for help. Remember that people, almost always, are so kind. I have often been overwhelmed by people seeing my distress and turning to help me.

Going on a longer journey – or anywhere new – by train or bus

Both require checking ahead of times and destination – but also an almost obsessive rechecking, because for me, even if everything is written down, I would forget, need to check, forget I had written it down… so a pen and notebook is vital for all the time information in a place where you can see it.

On Railway stations there is that need to constantly check the information boards... I found that very hard because they move – so for me looking at an information board with words disappearing, moving and reappearing to check destinations and times was extremely difficult. It was hard to actually see it, and then the movement made it hard. In addition, in many main Railway stations there are constant loud announcements. All of this can seem like an assault – almost impossible to actually remember or distinguish much of the information.

I learnt not to try to find my destination through these notice boards if possible. Usually I can find a person. And again I have experienced so much kindness and help when I ask for it.

I am going to give just one example from Birmingham New Street Station, which, as anyone who has been through it will know, is extremely busy, very noisy, and has lots of escalators up and down to numerous platforms. I have spent several hours there as part of changing trains. As soon as I arrived I would go and sit in a café, calmly, acclimatising to the movement and noise – until I felt ready to find someone to help me find the right platform. There is always someone. Often they would hand me over to someone else on the platform to make sure I got on the right train.

The process of working out where you are and what you are meant to be doing and how to get where you are going continues as you arrive somewhere. All the time. So the trick is to have the Survival bag so you can stop anywhere and be relatively warm and rest. To ask for help – and to know you may need to ask for help. To have ways to contact people, a list of what to do in case your brain crashes and you can't remember... taking yourself out as if you were a child, holding yourself by the hand. And finding that way to GROUND yourself, to bring a KIND attitude towards yourself. It is easy to be critical and think you should do better.

For me, more and more, these were times to use my Mindfulness Practices, even to just Notice you are upset, agitated, tired... and then to just allow yourself to acknowledge how that is and to

GROUND yourself.
Just become aware of the body, either feet on floor... maybe feet walking, or body sitting on a chair or a bench.
Noticing whatever the contact points are – and feeling them – the weight of the body. In contact with the ground or the seat.
And becoming aware of your breathing, just noticing and following as you breathe in and out. Nothing else to do. Just aware of being here. Of breathing. And then perhaps remembering whatever is going on, to think of yourself kindly. Ah, this is tough – I am tired – I don't know what to do... just

acknowledging whatever is here for you, and be kind as you might be to a child, or a loved other. And notice and allow the movement of your breath, in and out of the body.

Chapter 24: And Change Goes Ever On and On

For age is opportunity no less
Than youth itself, though in another dress,
And as the evening twilight fades away
The sky is filled with stars,
Invisible by day
(Henry Wandsworth Longfellow)

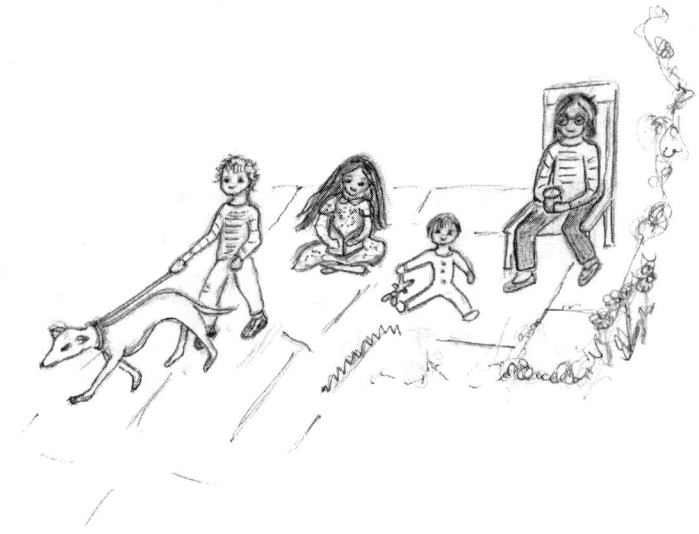

We never know, do we, where our journeys will take us?

The next couple of years go by, visiting my grandson N, who is riding along by the canal on his little scooter, loving to ride it into town to his favourite café for a babyccino – and now another baby was on its way. Later that year, J was born. So now I have my step-grandson R, who later on the same year gets married to P (both now at university), and my granddaughter A, and grandsons N and now J. I feel so grateful that I am still here to meet them all.

I felt established, I had become used to how I am – how I was, and I am OLD now. Perhaps it is always strange to find yourself old – not suddenly – it sort of grows with you. But maybe because I had been so taken up with recovery and illness, and in how my brain haemorrhages/strokes had changed me, and how I coped with it (putting down all the changes to the strokes), that I did not expect what came next.

There seemed to be even more changes in my head. I realised quite suddenly that, after years without, that I was Dreaming again when I went to sleep. I did not remember these dreams, as I had so often done before – but I knew when I woke up that my mind had been busy during the night.
That calm that had so often been with me was interrupted by periods now of quite high anxiety. I would wake feeling anxious without any particular cause. I found that I had lost some of the new found confidence in myself.

Most distressing of all was that my memory had changed. It was always scattered since the Tsunami, which was now seven years ago, but now the pattern of my thinking seemed different and there was a new sensation inside my head.

Sometimes it was busier, but in an anxious sort of way. It was more active than it had been for years. I noticed on the long walks that I would go on most days with my dog – where before I had been aware of a calmness, an awareness of my surroundings, each tree, the leaves, the feel of the breeze on my face – now often became full of jumbled memories and vague anxieties.

My memory changed, I FELT it. It had never been good since that first stroke, but I had got used to it – and to compensating, making recordings of thoughts as they came, making notes, letting go. But now it began to feel as if great slabs of thought and memory were dropping in chunks from my Mind – far more intensely than before. It was as if they were never to return. There was a finality to this. I found it harder to record things and if I did, I didn't know where, so my notes lay scattered around me. I could see my thoughts and memories go tumbling away, to lie scattered around me, or sometimes to seem to melt into a pool of nothing, a blankness. And with this was a worry, what was I thinking? What was I doing? There was a knowing that something had gone.

My sleep changed too. One of the things I mentioned before that I had noticed from the beginning was how deeply I seemed to sleep, and that I did not seem to dream at all – or if I did it was below any conscious remembering. I had noticed this particularly because it was a loss for me. I had had quite vivid dreams ever since being a small child, and I remembered dreams from far back – waking in my Nursery and looking through the bars of my cot. Throughout childhood, at my Boarding Schools, I dreamt vividly, often remembering the story themes and the times of nightmares. And years later when I worked as a Psychotherapist, I became interested in the meanings of dreams in a different way. Dreaming had been an important ever-present part of me.

They had stopped with the Tsunami – that first Brain Haemorrhage. But now they were back, in a different form, it seemed. I did not notice stories but had more of a sense of jumbled activity; I knew I had been dreaming but not of what.

And at this time I also became aware that my memory was even worse. And this became most obvious to me when I was working.

Ending my work as a teacher and therapist

Since I had left the Mindfulness Centre as Director, I had continued to teach Mindfulness – working with my colleagues. I taught courses on how to teach and understand Mindfulness-Based Approaches, and also ran residential Mindfulness Practice Retreats. Alongside that, I began to return to my work as a Psychotherapist, resuming a Psychotherapy practice even if much reduced. I also continued to work as a Supervisor of practitioners who used Mindfulness as a part of their work as Counsellors or Therapists. This was very much as I used to do, just greatly reduced. Much of my Supervision work was over the phone. Over these next years, this was very privileged and precious work for me, supporting others in their work with mindfulness – as teachers, therapists, supervisors and in their own practice.

I was able to write, far more slowly and deliberately than before, but I found my attention had changed and I could only write for half an hour at a time – whereas before I would have carried on for hours. I published articles and two Book Chapters on Mindfulness and Individual Therapy, one jointly written with Frances Larkin,[1] a colleague, psychotherapist and mindfulness teacher. I felt I was BACK. I could still do this work, and I loved it and loved working with all the wonderful people I was privileged to work with.

Yet all of this seemed to be changing. Before, I could remember the content of sessions, with some help from note taking – what people had told me, the theme of our work together, the dates and times of our appointments – now, by 2017, this began to change, to drop away.

My dear friends and colleagues saw the changes, and we devised ways of allocating pieces of teaching for me in a way that I could manage. In order to prompt my memory, I just needed to know WHAT I was teaching, rather like we need to know to open a book at the right chapter. But more and more as time went on, I didn't seem to know what chapter we were on. I could lose it in the middle of something. I would know it had gone. There were these moments of thinking 'What are we doing? What just happened? What did I just say?' – they became more frequent.

---

[1] Mardula, J. & Larkin, F. (2014) Mindfulness in Individual Therapy. In Dryden, W. & Reeves, A. (Eds). The Handbook for Individual Therapy (sixth edition, Pp.445-468). London, SAGE.

Chapter 24: And Change Goes Ever On and On

One of the beauties of Mindfulness is to notice what goes on in the Now, in THIS moment. That meant that I was good at noticing and knowing what's going on, knowing that I had lost direction – there is a feeling in the brain and in the body. So I knew what was going on NOW, in these moments, and I could feel the shift and see things as they slipped away.

Later, they fell faster, as if great chunks of ice were melting and breaking away to fall into the sea of everyday life around me. Sometimes I could see them floating away, or perhaps just lying there, beside me. At first I could name them, but I couldn't grasp them (you can't pick up ice or water).

I didn't try to hide it. That too was helped by the nature of my work, and by my Mindfulness practice. It was also what we were actually teaching – becoming aware of whatever is happening for each of us right now, in this present moment. And to notice whether it is Pleasant or Unpleasant, or if maybe we are indifferent to the experience. We taught and learnt through theory and personal meditation to become aware of what is happening, whatever it is, and to accept that it is there.

As the year progressed, the changes continued. In many ways I was working more deeply, more effectively with people. I could be very present with individuals, a group or a class in that moment, and in those moments of teaching, or particularly with therapy, deeply listening. But also, I began to know that I was not remembering. I was forgetting what had happened. Although, interestingly, I never forgot the content, or the emotion of moments, I did begin to forget the story or the subject of something. I knew that it was time to stop this work. I didn't have to disappear, we could talk about it, how that was for people, gradually closing and make transitions where necessary.

My process of gradually becoming less and less aware of time, and sometimes what had just happened, increased. It was a little similar to how I had been right back there at the start of this journey, when I first went out and about on the Bus. I noticed that even in daily tasks and events, it became difficult to manage time – and sometimes to remember the content of what was happening.

Gradually daily tasks which I had relearnt, such as food shopping, remembering I needed to put diesel in the car – and then – quite distressingly, although also with some humour – HOW to put the diesel in the car.

I had realised on my way to shop in Tesco one day that I was nearly out of fuel so I turned into the Tesco garage – to find that it was very crowded and I was in a queue. Then, when I finally got out at the pump, I was confronted by having not just to put the fuel in but having to press various keypad combinations to choose the fuel, how much fuel, how I would pay etc, and my card details. (I was learning that this was one of the worst situations for me to find myself in, because it requires organisational and sequencing skills, which for me now were in short supply.) I could do it, I told myself – but I felt my brain slipping and crashing. I stood and stared at the machine, panicking as a cacophony of hoots and shouts came from the long queue behind me. Someone shouted for me to hurry up.

But once again I was so struck by the kindness of people. I felt like crying or running away, neither of which would have been much help! So I went to the woman in the car directly behind me and said, 'please can you help me, my brain has crashed... I just can't do this'. She immediately got out, turned around and shouted at the irate people behind to stop it, and calmly got the information she needed from me, did it all, put the diesel in, and told me to drive over to the side and park, and she would come in and help me pay. And that is what she did. I managed to drive – rather shaken in my confidence, I think, which is so unlike me, even the brain injured me. Then I went and sat in the café for quite a while before doing the shopping.

And I have described this in some detail, because as I now know this sort of thing can happen at any time. It happens to most of us, brain injured or not, and the quality of it with Brain Injury is just more frequent and maybe a bit harder to come back from. It just needs me to be a little bit tired and for some unforeseen thing to arise – and I crash. This is common, to brain injuries, to anyone who is recovering from shock or illness, and of course to ageing. I have learned not exactly to expect something like that to happen, but to know that it might. It is then not a shock when it happens, and I have built up some ways which help me to deal with the slipping mind and stumbling brain.

At this time I went back to the Brain Injury Clinic for another set of Cognitive Tests – the results were much as before, but there was a change in my memory. They suggested that it might be helpful for me to go to the Memory Clinic for some tests on my memory, and also they would send me for a scan.

I was very resistant to this – I knew what they were looking for, whether I had the beginnings of Dementia. I had just spent over six years recovering from the Haemorrhages. It had been a hard slog in many ways, but I had built my life up again. I had learnt to shop, drive and organise my life. I could even manage the occasional loud cinema. I had begun to write this book, paint again, walk further with my dog each day, go to exhibitions, play with and look after my grandchildren. I had had enough, I would not go. There was nothing wrong with me – I had a Brain Injury, not Dementia.

And then, reading some of the wonderful Mindfulness and Buddhist books and the poetry that I had gathered and been sent by dear people over the years, I turned to my Meditation Practice. What we term as 'turning to the

Cushion'. And I took all this turmoil to my mindfulness practice. Such a wonderful resource. And each day I sat for 20 minutes. And you might like to do this with me:

SETTLING WITH DIFFICULTY PRACTICE

My intention was to sit, and breath and notice as best I could whatever was here, in my heart, body, in my mind, and to, as best I could, just be with that, whatever it was, breathing.
Taking my seat,
Adopting an upright posture,
Letting the eyes close and hands rest comfortably on the lap.
Becoming aware of the contact and weight of the body on the cushion or chair.
Becoming aware of the posture of the whole body, the weight going down and the height going up
The head reaching up toward the sky.
Watching and feeling the In Breath and the Out Breath.
Just sitting and Breathing.
This breath all the way in… this breath all the way out
And if the Mind wanders off as minds do,
Just coming back to the Body sitting here
And the Breath moving In, moving Out.
And as we sit we may notice thoughts and feelings come up
So not trying to do anything with then,
Not hanging on or pushing away.
With an attitude of gentle kindness towards yourself
Just sitting and breathing.
*And if pain, or worrying thoughts, or **difficulty** arise in the body*
Then as best you can do not push them away or try to avoid them
But sit and breathe allowing even this to be here.
Sitting
Breathing
*This breath all the way in, breathing around or into the **difficulty***
And then letting go of whatever is here as you breath out.
And doing this for a few times, or however long is right for you.
And then coming back to attention on the weight of the body
The movement of the breath
And coming to the end of this practice.

Or I would, as I have so often done over these years, go on my daily walk with my dog – to the fields, to the beach, to my favourite little wooded park nearby.

WALKING MEDITATION

And when we walk we can always turn that into a Walking Meditation – simply bringing attention to the fact that we are walking:

Noticing that I am walking
Being curious and noticing how that feels in the body.
Becoming aware of the contact of each foot as it rests on the ground
And then noticing how we pick the foot up and the weight shifts to the other foot.
Just walking, this step... this step... attention fixed on the sensation of moving the feet and them resting on the ground.
And becoming aware of the movement of the breath as we walk,
This breath in... this breath out.
Maybe breathing into the feet as they move
This step... breathing. This step... breathing.
And if the attention wanders off and you realise you have moved away from attention on the feet... then congratulate yourself for noticing, for becoming aware... and simply bring the attention back to the feet – this breath – this step – this breath...
Until you finish and come out of this practice and carry on with your day.

This is ALWAYS here – as long as we have breath we can breathe in and out and notice, feel our weight against the earth. And I would, as I had done from the beginning, recite to myself one of my remembered poems.

Only those wonderful poems, that I had been so thrilled, so grateful that I had been able to recite, to hold in my memory – to hold in my body almost as if I had eaten them – had gone: not completely, now and then one would be there, but I had lost my poems as an immediate resource, and that scared me and distressed me.

So I sat, as I do when distressed, and meditated. Then I felt the need to write this down, this story, and that helped me to let go of wanting things to be different again. How easily we go back into railing against how things are, but that way lies suffering.

Yes, something was happening in my brain. I knew it, and I would accept that it was there, whatever it was, This Too, This Too, with kindness and compassion and curiosity, those twin gifts of Mindfulness... not to choose to suffer and want things to be different – but to turn towards and be with whatever was here now, just as I had back there on the hospital trolley that became my Raft.

Neuro Notes 6: Relationships and Family Care

It is entirely natural to want a loved one to be the same as they were before their stroke or brain injury, and, as Jody has pointed out, being 'the same' again is the yardstick we often use to measure 'recovery'. It can be very hard for family and friends to be with someone who has changed as a person.

It can be difficult to look after someone while trying to be their partner or their son or daughter at the same time – particularly so if the relative has changed as a person.

Looking after someone with disabilities or who has changed as a person can be very demanding and stressful. Family caregivers often don't have the time or energy to take time out for themselves or to relax. They may feel that the stroke or brain injury has taken over their life as well as their relative's. Family carers need to look after themselves too.

Depression and anxiety are both very common among family caregivers. They often need support from outside to help them cope with their role and to keep going.

People often feel isolated and rather alone after a stroke or brain injury. This happens especially if they have had to leave work, or cannot take part in social activities as they used to. It helps some families to join a stroke or head injury group, to meet others with similar experiences. The injured person may feel they have something more valuable to offer here, and most people feel better and less isolated when they talk to others who are 'in the same boat'.

Families often benefit from understanding more about stroke or brain injury, from sharing their experiences with other families and from regular 'time out' opportunities to do something entirely for themselves.

Part 7: Leaving the Camp

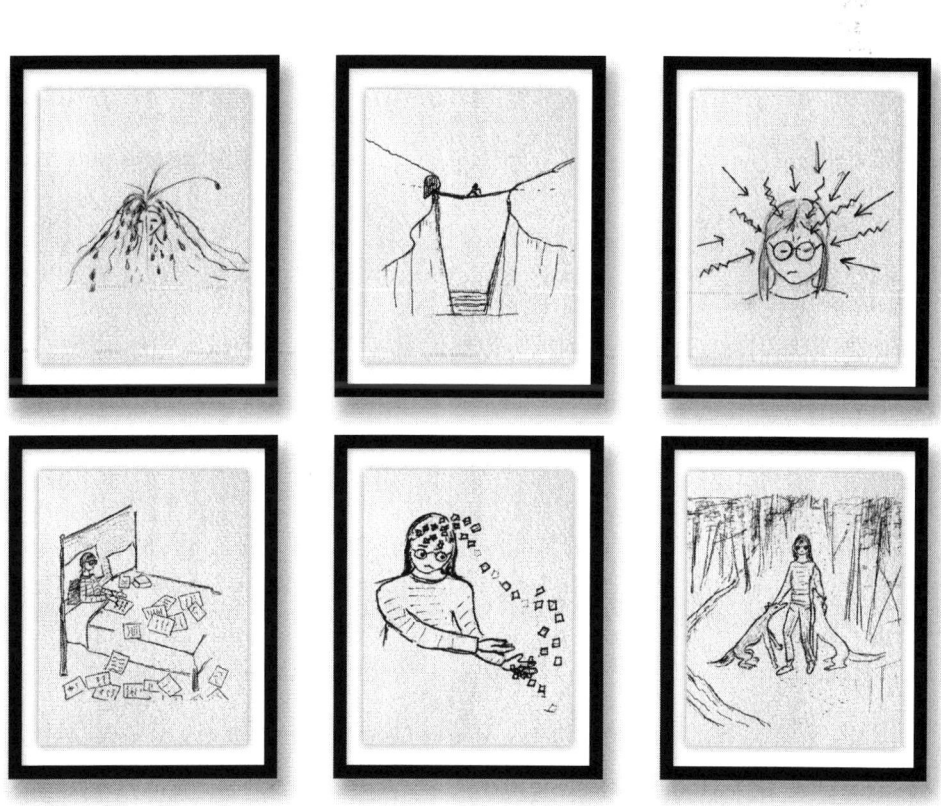

Chapter 25: Memory Clinic and Tattoo

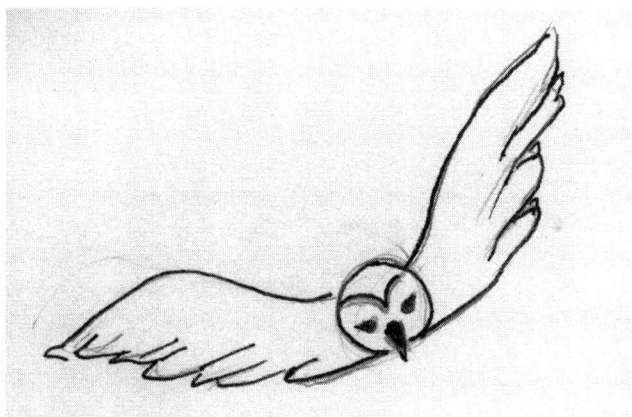

I had been going to the Brain Injury clinic on and off for five years but now I was referred to the Memory Clinic.

The very wonderful clinical neuropsychologist at the Brain Injury Clinic, who worked with me, sat with me and listened patiently for many hours drawing the information out of me – I was and am hugely grateful to her, and indeed all those who worked with me in those early years after the Tsunami. She carried out tests and explained to me what had happened to my brain and how it would affect me, and helped me to come to terms with that. The emphasis of my learning was on what had happened to my brain and to understand why it felt a certain way – what difficulties and differences there were. This is incredibly important, to understand and normalise the changes.

All this had helped me make the changes in my life that supported how I was now.

But now I was going for an assessment to the Memory Clinic, and, as I had known was possible, they diagnosed me with Vascular Dementia.

The style and atmosphere of the Memory Clinic is very different to the Brain Injury Service which is quite bare and clinical. The Memory Clinic is quite homely, and more informal. The emphasis is less on testing and questioning, and more on listening and explaining.

They too start with a questionnaire, but much shorter. Their emphasis seemed to be more on information about everyday living and behaviour, rather than on my thinking processes. But whereas the cognitive work at the Brain Injury Clinic helped me to understand WHY I was as I was, the Memory Clinic seemed to have a stronger element of responding to HOW I was. There is a very different outcome, I suppose.

With my Brain Injury I was then learning to live and cope and build new skills, to return to living my life as fully as possible. With Dementia I was learning to accept and learn how to be with my deteriorating brain and accept the loss. There was no recovery from this.

I had learned ways to approach and work with the changes in my brain – how I walked, how long I did something for, what things like timetables, planning, relearning how to cook, drive, all of this was behavioural.

Dementia, on the other hand, was not as structured. That is because the brain itself, instead of having a changed structure, has a dissolving of structure – or that was how I understood it from the inside.

Memory was affected by the Brain Haemorrhage – but nowhere as much as I began to experience it now. A good example here is the writing of this book. I began to write a couple of years after the second Brain Haemorrhage. And although it was slow progress I always knew what I had written, which number chapter I was on, and what I wanted to write about next. I might get the pages and numbers muddled up, but I knew the content. I might repeat some of the content, but somehow I kept the whole in mind. In contrast to this, writing now, not long after receiving the Vascular Dementia diagnosis, I find I am increasingly muddled.

I know that if I go off to make a cup of tea, I need to make notes and make a trail of them or I will probably forget I was in the middle of writing something. Closing the PC down is fatal. It all just stops existing. It is very much a case of out of sight out of mind. I do still know the sequence of the first four parts of the book. I can see them in my mind's eye – this part, then this part, the chapters in Part 4 and 5. Now, I cannot hold them all in memory at one time. I am quite likely to wake up tomorrow not knowing I have written any of this. Unless I have left myself some notes, I could well start all over again.

I am going to stop now, I am tired, and I feel too tired to write a lot of notes. I will just put one note on top of the PC and one by the kettle in the kitchen saying 'you are typing a Chapter near the end'. When people say to me, 'oh we all do that', it is quite annoying! Yes we do, I have often done that – but it has an entirely different quality to the memory loss that is Dementia-led. I do not pick the reminder up with an immediate 'oh yes!' I do not immediately remember, although I do know I forget and welcome this reminder – but what Chapter am I on? Am I typing something? What is it?

Once again Mindfulness comes in, because I will often take the notes from yesterday, or earlier, and go and sit down on my meditation cushion with the reminders in front of me. Rather than trying to go into my cognitive mind, which does not seem to work very well, I breathe, and allow a space where – not always but often – I find I know what it was that I was doing. I have to write it down then. I am learning that even the slightest interruption can send it all off into oblivion once more.

It is as if I am having to learn to entirely trust and go with process – with what I am experiencing right now. Trust that what I need to know is here, even if I can't immediately bring it to mind. Grasping makes it retreat further, I think. So I breathe, open, and trust and stay calm – it will come, and if it does not, I will just go with whatever seems right in this moment.

I am finding this all a rather lovely way to be. It doesn't work so well if doing something with someone else, or with a group where some sort of norm of how and what we are doing needs to be established. But it works well for wandering through each day on my own. The dog is not troubled by my random inconsistencies – as long as he gets fed and has his walks!

I discover a new way to record reminders. There were and are things I have worried about losing. Things I want to remember. Things that are useful to remember and that actually help me to structure life and retain memories. Because my Mindfulness Practice is so useful, and pleasurable, I hoped I would not lose it. I think perhaps because it is held more in the Body than the Brain it may well stay – time will tell. But I wanted to find a way to record the underpinning meanings behind the meditations. Buddhist teachings are often described in visual images and mandalas. So I decided to have a Tattoo.

This was an exciting adventure for me. There is a whole world of Tattoo images on the internet – and I enjoyed myself learning about them and choosing a traditional design that meant something for me. It is on my lower left arm – and is a circular design. It has a particular meaning that I am not going to describe here because that is not what it is for, although people often want to know what it is and why I have it. Its function is to physically remind me, by its visual presence as a part of my body. I enjoyed the process of having the Tattoo. It is a skilled art form and there is something beautiful in being the canvas. Everybody always asks did it hurt… and the answer is yes and no. I just find it such a comfort – always there, reminding me to stop, to breathe, to notice when my mind is judging or getting caught up in criticising or in anxious thoughts and fears. It is a reminder to notice when I do this, and to choose to stop and let go of the thoughts and to breathe – just to let go and come back to now. This moment, this breath, bringing in kindness and acceptance, even of this, even of this.

And I liked it so much, this constantly present visual teaching on my arm, that I had another, higher up my arm, of a Lotus flower. The Lotus has to grow through mud and darkness before blossoming above into a flower of impermanent beauty. We too go through dark times before we blossom in the light – and everything we experience, is impermanent, even ourselves. Then I had an Owl tattoo. She is on my shoulder – and is a symbol of seeing in the dark.

These companion symbols have been with me during this last year, and it has been a difficult year in many ways.

Chapter 26: The Unseen Wounds of Brain Injury

I have been writing this book for a long time now and in the process my sense of my aging has grown. At the time of my first brain injury I was 65, and now, as I draw it all together, I am 72 and physically more frail.

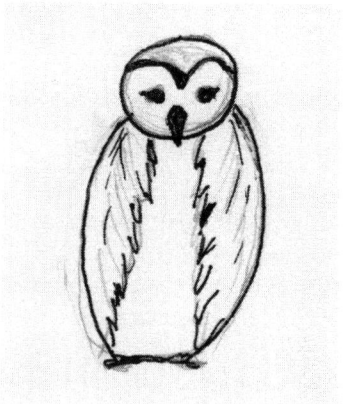

Writing this morning, I see that yesterday's snow flurries have hardened into sheets of ice. The combination of a frail and older body and the lack of balance that has been with me since the brain injuries traps me in my house.

I return always to my Mindfulness Practice, wondering for the hundredth time how I would have managed this recovery, and indeed life, without it.

My main hope in writing this book has been that others may also find this path, using an awareness of Mindfulness practices, of accepting and being able to just be with whatever is there in each moment – this path (in many ways a simple path) to finding peace within the losses. I am hoping that this book will support them in the pains and confusions that walk hand in hand with brain injury. And for those who watch and care for them, whose lives too have been turned around by the brain injuries of another.

In the chapter 'Wolves in the Woods', I came face-to-face with the Wolves of Love and Hate – what I want and what I don't want. Here I am again – despairing about the ice, wondering how I will get out, walk my dog, buy food, with my fear now of falling. I think back to the days when I was fully confident that my body and my mind would cope with any difficulty – certain I would know what to do about an icy path. Indeed, I would probably have cleared it myself, and known that I could take care as I walked on the icy bits.

As I have discovered again and again, it is the worry about things, and the wanting to get rid of or change things, that causes much of my unhappiness or dissatisfaction. Listening to the Wolf of Hate: 'Oh no, not this, I will fall, it will be awful, I can't cope – there is no one to help me', etc. And again I turn to my Mindfulness Practice and ask myself, 'what is going on now?'

I FEEL my Body sitting here.
I FEEL my weight on the chair and the floor.
I am aware of the tightening and tension in my body
As I think of falling.
My jaw tight – my shoulders hunched.
AND I SAY TO MYSELF the words of the Wolf of Love:
It's OK. Let go of the thoughts.
Let the tension go.
Let the shoulders and the jaw soften and relax.
Let the arms just rest comfortably.
Feel the contact of my feet on the ground.
And now I follow the In Breath and the Out Breath
This Breath All The Way In
This Breath All the Way Out
Just breathe this way for a while.
As thoughts come into my mind, just noticing them
And deliberately letting them go
Not getting caught up in them.
And turning towards a sense of comfort and gentleness
And opening without fear to planning the next stages of the day.

I know, as I choose to sit and breathe in this way, that I can let go of that tendency to focus on the worrying or frightening thoughts. I can connect with my own wisdom and confidence and know what to do with whatever is here – ice, snow, cold, confusion. I have this Mindfulness Practice (what I still think of as the Wolf of Love, whispering to me that all is well).

And after all these years, getting used to the changes my brain injury has brought... the losses, sometimes the gains, the friendships, kindnesses, my own intrepidness – as well as the loneliness, fears and isolation that have sometimes been here... I realise again that there is no getting better that means 'getting rid of' – that I can never go back.

But that I can stay in each moment with the gift of my Breath, that I do not have to suffer at the circumstances of my life. That this is what it means to be human.

THIS has been my particular path of learning.

To unite with my own particular Wolves of Love and Hate, I have learned to trust my own strengths – to learn how to stay with this moment now – to let go of journeying to places of fear – and thoughts of problems and difficulties. To rejoice – in just being me – in this beautiful world – however I am – with the contact with all the wonderful people I encounter.

What else can we do with our one life – our one world?

And I sit and wish you all well – all those affected in whatever way by Brain Injury and Stroke and Dementia – and all who are connected or care for someone who is.

Sometime later that morning I come downstairs to find that the ice has melted.

I am not trapped in the house after all. And I smile – all that suffering I gave myself for a while – the oh no – disaster – I will fall. It has all gone now.

All things change – move on... everything in my life is impermanent – how I was 'before', how I am 'now'.

My Brain Injury opened my eyes to the beauty to be found in the most unlikely places... the calm and peace to be found in the middle of what can seem the darkest times.

And also there are those Unseen Wounds – as I carry on, returning to what has become a New Normal life – there are many differences to how I am, and how I guess I would have been without having had the Brain Injuries.

And it seems important to name and know them. In a way, by acknowledging the distresses and difficulties that are here, it helps me to begin to accept them, and bring my Mindfulness Practice into how I respond. And the attitude, to be curious, to see if I can manage to live WITH this, as comfortably as possible, is much gentler. It is much kinder and more supportive to be like this than railing and fighting against it and wanting it to be different and go away.

I have my moments of anger and despair – and my practice then is often to go out – go to my woods. Rather than just walking and breathing, I STAMP my feet and remember to breathe and (if no one is around!) I might SHOUT something – of how upset, or confused, and irritated I am just then. Then I allow that to go – to go on the voice, and come back – 'No, I DON'T LIKE IT'. Sometimes, of course, I would love to be as I was before... AND also, this is how it is... This is how I am. And suddenly there is a different feel to my thoughts, my experience, how I feel in my body. And I walk and breathe and become aware of THIS moment, what is around me, what I will do today... Breathing, smiling – just the action of smiling can sometimes change a mood, I find.

And for me, it has been helpful to acknowledge the Unseen Wounds that are there – when they are shut off, hidden, they seem to have more power.

One thing I have found, and often been frustrated by, is that mostly the person with a brain injury tends not to be understood. Many people seem to want to believe that they are not as severely affected as in fact they are. They just want them to get better.

I wonder if people tend not to understand because they haven't got anything to relate it to?

They don't want to think of it, of what has happened and is happening to their loved one, their friend. When brains are damaged, it seems to be more frightening for others – maybe because it is about Identity – the Who and what and how the person is. It is often almost a loss of that person...

Maybe it is different with a physical illness, even very severe ones like cancers. Perhaps we can have an inkling of what it would be like to have a Cancer, or another serious and life threatening physical condition or injury. Maybe we can relate to the pain and physical problems the person might be experiencing. Even in losing a limb... the person involved stays the same loved person... but losing some of the brain, some of the personhood?

I would probably have been just the same before this happened to me – but I am not so sure that people can relate to what it's like to be confused and not be able to remember something. No, no, it won't come back. Others often come with their 'solutions' – their Post Its – their Notice Boards – their 'reminders on the phone' and note books and other ways to cope. It can be very isolating because there is no real understanding of how it is for you. All these coping techniques are fine, but they hardly touch the surface. They certainly are not a solution. There isn't a solution – but there is acceptance.

And sometimes I know people have got an inkling of what I am talking about – that I am referring to a COMPLETE change in how I am inside, and how I live with me in the world.

In some ways, it is frightening for others to sense this, I think, because it is almost like being on the edge of madness... when the brain functions differently. It is a completely different world, perspective and way, for me anyway, and for many others I talk to with Brain Injury. It is a completely different experience of being with and within this Me in the world. And that too is frightening.

But it is also EXCITING – and I think that is part of why have written this book. It is an EXCITING journey I have been on and am still on. It is a journey into the unknown, a journey of recovery that everyone can see. I don't use my stick so much now, but inside, INSIDE THE BRAIN, it IS different. It is a bit like my brain being like a broken leg but inside my mind... and it HASN'T

MENDED – it is functional, I can walk on it, but it HASN'T mended. No one can see it. No one wants to hear about it… they want to hear it is better or at least getting better. I am not so sure there is a 'better', because the change is so deep and is about your very being. I cannot 'use a stick' for my brain.

I really want people to get a sense of this – and perhaps see if we can REALLY listen to one another and what the Brain Injured person says, letting go of wanting to know about how it is better now – and what might help. Sometimes we just need to have HOW IT IS – however stark – HEARD and allowed to be spoken. And in THAT – the Being Heard – there is great healing. So my encouragement is to be curious, and interested, if you can.

How is it? How are You? And listen to the response and let them feel, yes, I am listened to… accepted. Maybe we can never be Understood – except by others that have walked the same path. Yet there is a healing in feeling understood – we will all know that.

We are all different. Everyone who goes through a Brain Injury goes through it on their own… It is a lonely path.

And each of us who have a brain injury, will bring our own package of life experience, our hopes, fears, strengths, weaknesses, knowledge, to our recovery.

I have had conversations with people who say that this is the same as being drunk – or being on drugs? I have done both in the past, and NO, it is not the same. I would have known 'I feel different because I have drunk something' etc… and in time I would go back to being 'me' again. Whereas now – there is NOTHING to go back to – that person is no longer here – there is no going back. I am me, the me I have always been BUT Changed, and we all have that need to be accepted just the way we are.

Chapter 27: A New Story to be Lived and Breathed

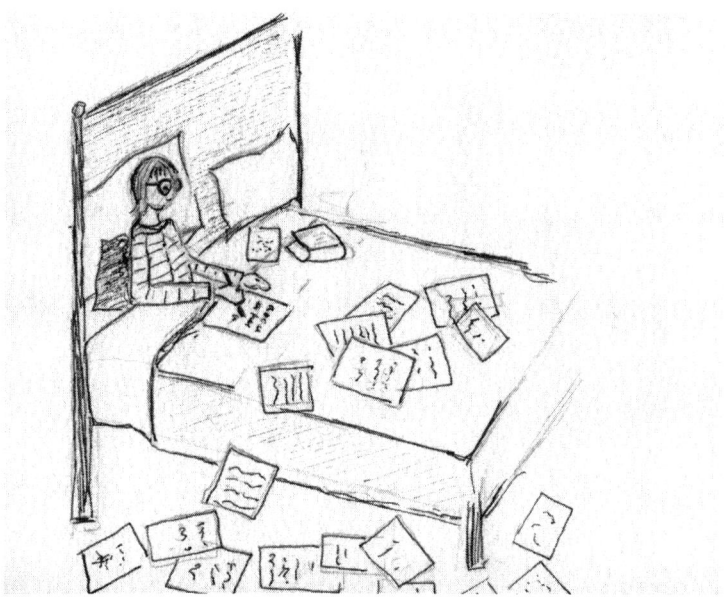

Allowing

So much seems to be falling now,
Falling from my head.
Piles of discarded
Writing, lie all around my bed.

Thoughts and plans and memories
What it was that was just said
Also join the growing pile
Growing around my bed

Strangely there are different mes
That watch things as they go,
As the light turns down on the here and now
Turns up on the long ago

But this is not a tale of woe,
Although change and loss are here,
It is a story about the OPENINGS
That appear when Loss is here.

Chapter 27: A New Story to be Lived and Breathed

It's a story about This moment,
This breath – This here – This now,
It's a story about curiosity
And how to be with – TO ALLOW.
(Jody Mardula)

It is very hard now to finish this book. It has been with me for so long – a companion of myself with myself.

I know now that one of the difficulties particularly common to Vascular Dementia is planning, and especially in following lists – sequences – numbering. They are all quite important in life, and certainly in structuring a book.

The content of all the chapters is here but I can spend ages, increasingly tired and distressed, trying to organise what I have just written and knowing (in one part of my brain) where it would go in the story, but also hating to force experience into the confines of chapters – the flow of the story suddenly truncated.

It is interesting… and I think clearly shows the sorts of problems that come with Vascular Dementia… and probably other Dementias too. As soon as one starts to put things into order, it doesn't seem to work. The plans, ideas, and the order sequence we want simply does not stay in the mind. It almost resists the attempt to order it and it falls away, resists and still lies there in a pile of muddle. All attempts at organising it themselves tumble away. Somehow it is hard to grasp and hold onto – thoughts – ideas – plans, follow directions. That organising and structured part of the brain does not seem to work.

A similar, and familiar process is going on for me now. I have just noticed that I am getting muddled and a bit stressed trying to write this last part of the book in the way I have written the rest of it. I don't seem able to pull out the memories and keep attention on them long enough to put it on paper… They do not seem to stay still – these recollections – they are fluid – as if I had thrown a stick into a stream and expected it to stay still… but it goes with the stream… and that may not be where I was going. It falls away.

Whatever has changed in my Dementia-influenced brain, it does not allow me to organise anything very much. Or to keep to a plan.

So I just continue randomly seeing what emerges. Writing this, I will just write – not plan. The organised story, whatever it was, has ended. I have entered a new place where time seems not to exist much and generally I am happy just pottering around in this moment. Wherever I may be – out and about, or mostly here in my house and garden, going on walks to my still familiar places… and smiling at the daily passing of familiar strangers faces.

I am aware of diary dates, people coming – occasional outings with family or friends, but I am alone most days with no particular structure. When I am with people, that seems to provide a structure. I feel more in control. I suppose there is some sort of inbuilt social learning on how to relate and BE WITH others which still kicks in. When I am alone, with just the dog, that structure seems to wobble. Sometimes, perhaps if there is a long gap alone, I feel myself more out of time – out of the structure of the world. The television and radio if I put them on, communication tools – they keep the structures going.

Other than the structure they provide, most days have no structure now... except this book – and when it is finished, I will notice the gap. This is not unpleasant – though I am aware it is necessary to keep some sort of structure. The practicalities of life – food, medicines – must all be continued. Having a dog ensures that bones are in good supply here! As is bird food – any major outings to shops always involve buying of bird seed and dog food.

Stopping driving – the car going – seemed to usher in another dip – the discipline of remembering how to drive. I am beginning to realise how important it is to hang on to structures. This was true to some extent with the Brain Injury – but there is a different quality to the absoluteness of Dementia perception – or at least as I experience it. If I was not writing this book I wonder if I would be so aware of this. Over these years of writing, I have developed a habit of observing – this sort of external observing of my process and experience. I think, too, that my ongoing Mindfulness Practice has played and does play a huge part in this. Being Mindful IS about being aware of this moment, turning towards ourselves with Kindness and Curiosity, and observing what our experience is in that moment. And so I am mindfully demented – I like that – because this is just another part of life – experienced... like most things... by some and not all. We are frightened of it – at least I never remember hearing dementia talked about in any sort of positive way, I don't think.

So here I am. Sitting on the edges now of this new Dementia phase. As with everything, I do not know what it will bring.

The Now world includes diary dates, people coming, occasional outings with family or friends – but most days have no particular structure. In the Now world dear colleagues come and help me with the book – my family make sure I organise shopping, have paid the bills and if there are any appointments I need to attend.

I look at the similarities and differences between my experience of my particular Brain Injuries and Dementia. I think I have reflected in different ways over the Brain Injured years on the impact of the changes in me on others. A lot of it was about behaviour, I think... and there is something different about Dementia – the differences in behaviour and more strongly in identity – in being.

But what is common between them, although felt increasingly frequently now, is confusion and utter, utter exhaustion.

Now – just remembering what I was planning and thinking about has become even harder. Generally I am better earlier in the day, but certainly my memory and planning deteriorates as the day goes on, even if I rest.

It helps if I write things down, but then I need to remember where it is – and even that I wrote something down. These tasks seem to get more difficult – many things can get in the way of remembering.

The simplest thing seems to bring on exhaustion. Certainly my level of fatigue has increased. I plan for that, make allowances... but any journey out, however well planned, seems draining. I imagine that my brain simply does not deal with different situations. Even regular tasks like getting on the familiar bus to go to the Doctor's surgery, which is only a 10-minute journey, can be enough to crash my brain. It is as if I just ran a couple of miles!

I notice too that a high level of fatigue will also affect my memory, so that things can just drop away. I simply do not know where I am for a while, or what just happened. And a lot of energy goes into recovering from that. Where am I? What just happened? What do I need to do now? I ask myself these questions, and go through a process. Generally I will then find a quiet place to sit for a while, if I can. Bus stop benches are good, benches and cafés if there are any nearby.

And if there is nowhere to stop and rest, then I walk, slowly, for a while. And whether sitting, in a private or public space, or walking, I turn to my Practice – and always as soon as I deliberately feel my feet on the ground, and notice the breath moving in and out of my body, there is a settling... and then gradually my mind clears.

Recently I have developed a new way of beginning a Mindfulness meditation. Most of the practices we use tend to give directions as to what to do – just as I have in the practices in this book. I may start with: Bring your attention to the breath, now follow the breath in and out... But more recently, perhaps as my brain slows and gets even more muddled, I cannot even always follow these simple directions. And by chance really, I discovered one day another way of guiding myself in and into a Practice.

Putting my hands in my coat pocket one day, standing in rather a noisy bus station – with loud announcements, a lot of noise around me – I found my brain, already wrestling with information about times and different buses, beginning to crash. Immediately I turned to my practice but found it hard to centre, and to bring my mind to attend to my body and my breath. This was a shock – as it is something I have always been able to do – almost automatically. I have taught so many others to do this. But in that moment, I felt something in my pocket. It was soft – I knew what it was – It was a small, soft baby toy owl that I must have put there when playing with one of my little grandsons… I held it in my hand and squeezed it. Just feeling that squeezing in and then letting go, I found I could direct my attention to the sensation of squeezing and then the feel of loosening my hold on the little soft owl… and I began to breathe. Noticing the inbreath as I felt the pressure of my hand squeezing the toy and then the outbreath as I released… and rather than trying to force my over tired, rather damaged brain to think In breath, out breath, somehow my hand was doing it for me. Squeezing and breathing in, releasing and breathing out. I didn't seem to have to think about directing the hand to squeeze and release, it just seemed like a natural thing to do.

Since I discovered this, I always have some soft object with me in my pocket. It could be a soft cloth ball, or any other object that can just comfortably fit in a pocket and be held in the hand (baby toys and dog toys are good for this). And when I simply hold that object and squeeze it, it seems to direct me to follow my breath. The contact with the soft toy reminds me to feel the connection of my feet on the ground or my body on the chair, meditation cushion, or bed. So the practice is led not by my tired brain, but kinaesthetically, by the sensation in my hand.

This hand-directed practice has become such a useful way to bring mindful awareness of each moment into my mind. Whether I am lying down, or sitting, or walking – there is no need to remember any sequence, and instructions, I can just respond to the sense of squeezing and releasing my hand, and follow the sensation of my inbreath and my outbreath.

There are many different ways that we can remind ourselves to practice… sitting, or walking or lying down and directing our attention to the body and the breath, following instructions for different meditation practices.

But they do require a level of organisation of thought – until perhaps we get so accustomed that we can direct our attention to our breath as soon as we think of it.

But the injured brain can sometimes benefit by having something that relies less on Intention… and arises more from sensation – like the sensation of movement in the hand and the connection to the movement of the breath.

I like that this practice is so very personal – We can choose an object that in itself has meaning for us – perhaps, as this external link to bring us back, back into the experience of being here now, in this moment, breathing – and that is what meditating is all about. Any soft, hand-sized object will do. It simply has to move like the breath, in and out.

However confused, tired and unwell we may be, there is always the breath to return to.

Chapter 28: Return to the Beginning

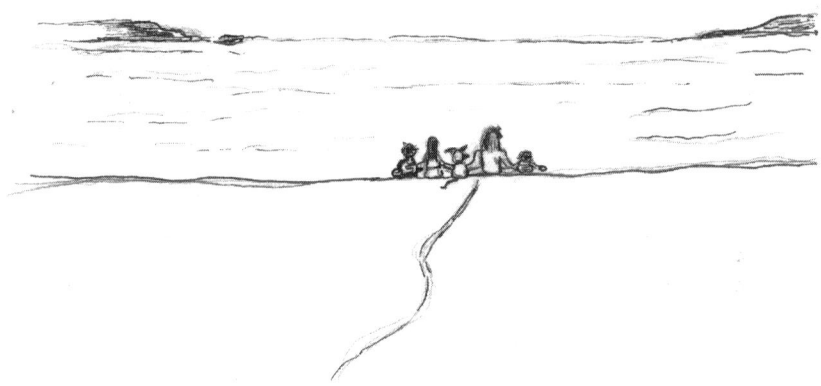

My great learning is that there is no such thing as recovery – if that means getting back to how I was before that first Haemorrhage. Instead, perhaps it is more about Discovery – Curiosity – and Acceptance of how I am now.

This seems to be a shared expectation – you are ill – you get better – and you are as you were before, you 'recover'. If there is a physical injury, something people can see, we seem better able to accept there may be changes. But changes in personality and our inner sense of self, of who we are, seem harder for us to understand and accept. Perhaps because it is unseen, there are no observable scars.

I am thinking of other illnesses, injuries I have had during my life, and how they may have marked me. Childhood illnesses – chickenpox, mumps, measles… they marked me with learning, the experience of being with itching, of wanting that to go away. Learning that things could not be just magicked away, even by powerful grown-ups – but with some early patience, left with just the fading memories and perhaps a few white small scars to mark their passing.

With a few minor breaks and fracture of arms there is pain, discomfort and itching of plaster casts. I remember being proud of my plaster cast when I fell off a horse and the pride of friends writing their name on it! It gave me a sort of status and importance.

Later, as a woman, there was the pain of childbirth. There were operations, some more serious than others, which brought changes to my body. There was learning from these experiences but none brought any essential changes to who I am, to my sense of self, in the way that Brain Injury has. Through arm injury, liver injury, back injury and others, I remained essentially the same. Some illnesses and injuries have carried their marks. Some periods of emotional upheaval and great distress have also – low times, sad times, all the ills and hurts and disappointments accompany each of us on our human journey.

Some physical and some emotional, missing out on a holiday, a job, a longed for treat. These become part of the fabric of our lives at different ages and stages, helping us learn how to deal with disappointment, loss, changed physical abilities – finding our way to recover and move on.

I later learned to see through Mindfulness eyes that I 'suffer' and increase that suffering when I want things to change, and to be different to how they are.

The consequences that would arise from the choices I made, the behaviours I engaged in, the stuff of all our lives changed as I grew. I changed as we all do – making mistakes, traversing the ups and downs of life, the joys, the tragedies, the gifts and losses of any life.

My Mindfulness practice over these last years has helped me find a path through the pain and difficulty, to find a new way to be with my experiences whatever they were, pleasant or unpleasant, without trying to change them or push them away.

And through all these life events, I stayed essentially the same ME – the same person I had always been, child, teenager, professional, mother... with all my strengths and faults. I spent many years learning my craft first as a Secretary, then Psychotherapist, Addictions specialist, then Mindfulness Teacher, Lecturer and as a writer. I was 'me'. 'Jody.'

The Brain Haemorrhages washed much of that away. I was indeed left like seaweed on the rocks, some lying there still clinging to the rock, and some washed out to sea or drifting on the tide before being swept up onto some unfamiliar shore. My knowledge and my memories scattered...

I was left with many 'anchors' to what I had before (although many gone for good and many fuzzy, hard to grasp, out of focus). But the memories were there, emerging from time to time, triggered by whatever was happening, from friendships, relationships, memories of work, of home, of this house and this village.

Yet somehow I now felt like a ghost walking in these familiar places.

Ghost

I walked the paths I walked before
Though not alone now anymore
Beside me I can hear and see
The ghost of who I used to be
I see her footprints in the sand
And reaching out, I hold her hand
It's sometimes her that others see
For them the ghost is the new me
She helped me learn to walk, to see
This person that I used to be
Who walks now side by side with me
(Jody Mardula)

And I realised I walk beside me, and the Me is this New Person, the one who is walking beside me is the ghost of who I used to be.

My Recovery has been something we acknowledge with each other. I have stopped trying to be one or the other – or, as expected, 'get back to normal', to be essentially how I was before. This IS the New Normal… this IS the community of the New Normal, the Brain Injured, The one now with Dementia. I see myself as having been on a journey of discovery that is still unfolding…

I cannot go back because the old me was indeed washed away by the blood tsunami swirling through every nook and cranny of my brain. That ME is not there to go back to. Over these 'recovery' years, where I thought I was travelling forward back to being the old Me, she was there all along – but now she walks hand in hand with the Me I am now.

I wonder why it has taken me so long to discover that? To let go of wanting things to return to how they were?

Maybe if I had been younger when I had those two bleeds, I would have taken a different path. But the New Normal began nine years ago with the first bleed when I was 65 (although of course I did not know it then) and has walked hand in hand with me along with the changes, some normal, some due to ageing.

But now, after this long slow writing, as I get ready to publish, nine years have passed and I am 74. As we age, our perceptions change anyway – as they do at all stages of life. Our outer world is perceived and viewed through our inner experience, life events and expectations.

Through my brain injury, I have had to develop 'new eyes', to learn to accept this New Normal I live in.

Chapter 28: Return to the Beginning

This is MY journey. I cannot know what journey others with Brain Injuries go on, but I do feel it will be a journey – and that those who are left behind, those who love us, often wait for the person we were before to emerge. Or maybe they try to push away the new changes – that often our love may make us yearn to have the old person back. And these changes may make us 'difficult' to be with, challenging in some ways, perhaps... I know I have been (probably still am).

All those who knew me also had to journey over the rope bridge to the new land. They have been willing to take this journey of discovery with me, although maybe they did not know we were on a life trek, not just a short path back to where we started!

It is a demanding role for our carers, friends and loved ones. At other times people are calling to me from the old world – the world across the rope bridge – wanting and waiting for me to come back. Some have not been able to travel here. They haven't let go... to see me as I am now... still waiting for the old me.

Over those first few post-haemorrhage years I noticed and recorded my experience in terms of leaving the old world, crossing the rope bridge and travelling over the plain to the mountain range... and as I came down from the mountains, there was a sense of being over the obstacles. Then the second haemorrhage struck me down.

But it is not the end yet – perhaps it never is. There is another journey, again unexpected, for me to take. Now with Vascular Dementia – the words I have dreaded hearing said – 'you have Dementia', I was told. But somehow I feel I have been on a long journey preparing and coaching me for this. Almost an apprenticeship.

It is a new journey. I don't yet know whether I will meet more wolves on the way, but there will be different challenges. Or maybe as Annee says in her lovely poem 'Compass', 'there are no wolves here, only foxes'.

My learning from these years of living with a damaged brain, of learning and developing a stronger Mindful attitude to life, sustained by Mindfulness Meditation, is of the love and support of friends and family, of learning the wonder of New Eyes which I open every day – and that whatever else goes on, whatever difficulties arise – I will be with this too. In the end we only ever have this one moment – this breath now... that is all we have to be.

I sat down to write my story, and as I did, I drew a map to chart my journey from my familiar, busy life, left behind as I travelled over the rope bridge, towards and over the mountains then the woods. And I found to my surprise that the path that seemed so long – it has been nine years – came out of the wood quite close to the coast.

I AM AT THE END OF THIS BOOK NOW… but so reluctant to let it go – to end. What an amazing adventure it has been – and of course still is. I remember as a child I so much wanted to go on adventures like the children in the books that were read to me and later I read myself. Rupert Bear Adventures, Famous Five adventures – later, books like Treasure Island and Kidnapped… perhaps these were all in mind as I visualised and experienced myself travelling over the rope bridge, the mountains, through the forests to the adventures of the Camp.

The capacity of our brains to tell stories – the gift of imagination – is still here, if different. Those early childhood books have helped me see life as an adventure – and I am grateful for that. It has allowed me to feel a part of my experience, to make choices as to how to live my life. I was not confined by the Brain Injuries and nor am I now confined by the Dementia – which comes and goes in waves at the moment – because I can't be. Perhaps the landscape will be less familiar than on my journey so far… maybe there are dark woods and wolves ahead… but I journey on… with curiosity… and that wonderful resource of the Breath. Turning to the Breath – the feet on the ground, or body sitting or lying here – and Breathing – there is only THIS MOMENT – and then THIS MOMENT… knowing that many others travel with me in these landscapes of the injured and changing brain. We are never alone. Every time someone new reads this book, we with our damaged and changing brains know that we walk alongside them – as they, our companions, whoever they are, join us on our journeying… Welcome.

PRACTICE

As we reach the end of this book together
PAUSING for a moment to feel
The weight of the body sitting here.
The contact of the body
with whatever is supporting it.
Bringing our attention to the breath…
… Following the movement
of the In Breath and the Out Breath.
This Breath all the way in.
This Breath all the way out.
Feeling the air on the lips
Feeling the rise and fall of the belly.
And Breathing in Love
Thoughts of love for ourselves
Thoughts of love for others
Of Kindness and Acceptance…
May all beings be well
May all beings be safe,
May all beings be happy.

All Things Pass

All things pass
A sunrise does not last all morning
All things pass
A cloudburst does not last all day
All things pass
Nor a sunset all night
What always changes?

Earth... sky... thunder...
mountain... water...
wind... fire... lake...

These change
And if these do not last

Do man's visions last?
Do man's illusions?

Take things as they come.

All things pass.
(Lao Tsu)

Neuro Notes 7: Vascular Dementia

Within the last year of writing this book, Jody discovered that she also has vascular dementia. The changes were mild at first, and have developed gradually. The dementia seems to have made Jody's stroke-related difficulties worse, particularly her memory problems.

The main difference between a stroke and dementia is that the stroke tends to improve over time, whereas dementia becomes slowly worse. It is often difficult to pinpoint exactly when or how the changes began.

Alzheimer's disease is the most common type of dementia, and after that, vascular dementia. Many people have a mixture of Alzheimer's disease and vascular dementia.

Alzheimer's disease causes chemical changes in the brain that interfere with its normal function. The substances that pass signals from one brain cell to the next are in short supply. There is also a build-up of abnormal proteins, which slowly destroy the brain tissue. Memory problems are usually the first sign of Alzheimer's disease, as it usually begins in areas that control memory.

Vascular dementia has less predictable effects. It is often caused by a series of small ischaemic strokes. These can occur in any part of the brain, and so the symptoms and changes have no fixed pattern.

An ischaemic stroke happens when a blood clot blocks the blood supply to part of the brain. Brain cells cannot survive if they are starved of oxygen and food for more than a few minutes. Each small stroke affects another small area of brain tissue, causing changes in memory, concentration and thinking that build up over time.

People with vascular dementia often become worse suddenly, when they have one or more small strokes, and then remain stable for a while. Jody feels that her strokes come in clusters – she is aware of several within a few days, and then they stop until the next cluster.

Memory problems are very common, as well as difficulties with concentration, planning and organisation; doing things in sequence; and visual perception. All of these difficulties overlap with the effects of Jody's stroke.

Memory and other cognitive problems become progressively worse over time. Later stages of dementia involve changes in emotion and behaviour too.

Changes in emotion and behaviour are usually mild at first and become more severe over time. Again, it can be difficult to remember when they started. No two people with dementia are alike – the kinds of change and how severe they are varies enormously from person to person.

Many different things can change – but no one person will have all possible problems.

Memory and attention problems can increase risk to the person as they struggle to maintain their independence – issues around driving, managing medication, setting fire to things when cooking, and getting lost are all very common. The person may not see the risks or the need for care and support. This transition towards greater dependence is often very difficult.

There can be issues around drinking enough fluids, medication, and personal hygiene routines – the person may insist that they had a bath this morning and refuse to have 'another one'. Situations like this can trigger dramatic mood swings, or there may be consistent personality changes, which can be difficult.

continued >

Sleep patterns often change; people with dementia are often up and about at night. The darkness and absence of people can add to existing confusion. 'Sundowning' is common in the middle stages – people become restless or confused as the light fades. In later stages, people may not know where they are or recognise their relatives, and may leave to try and find their way home.

People can be afraid, suspicious or even paranoid. The person may move their belongings or hide them, but then forget where they are and accuse others of stealing them. People with Alzheimer's Disease, in particular, are often not aware of their memory problems and other difficulties.

Susan McCurry's book *When a Family Member has Dementia: Steps to becoming a resilient caregiver* is one of many helpful resources available in this area. She describes some compassionate strategies that can help to prevent difficulties, and solve problems when they arise.

Jody's Experience of Dementia

In recent conversations about her dementia, Jody told me that it feels very different to the stroke. Her memories are being 'rubbed out' rather than falling away or slipping. Whilst we were talking, Jody drew some pictures of herself. A giant rubber was gradually deleting parts of her – memories, abilities and personality.

Jody was accepting of the dementia diagnosis in the beginning, but as her difficulties have become more pronounced, her attitude has wavered. Some days she is more anxious generally, and more concerned about the future. Jody is more tired now, but still feels very resistant to having any help.

Jody's memory has good days and bad days. Things are not consistent and this is difficult for other people to understand. Jody is often aware of her difficulties; people with vascular dementia tend to have more insight than people with Alzheimer's disease.

Jody has noticed that people are often uncomfortable when they realise that she is confused or has forgotten something – perhaps because they do not know what to say. Understandably, not everyone has the confidence to remind Jody about what she has forgotten.

Conversations with Jody continue to be very lively. She is insightful, amusing, and able to remember many things – although she often forgets what we said ten minutes ago.

We tend to assume that if a person can't remember things, or if they become overwhelmed or confused, their other faculties and abilities will be unreliable too. Jody's experience suggests that the opposite is true.

Jody is aware of further changes in relationships. She feels she may be more difficult to be with now. She has lost confidence in how she comes across to people – she may look cross when she is just struggling to explain something.

She is more sensitive to things that trigger old emotional issues – they are closer to the surface now.

A Personal Perspective

My mother died last year at the age of 96, after living with dementia for more than ten years. She almost certainly had a mixture of Alzheimer's disease and vascular dementia. She lived next door to my sister, which allowed her three daughters (but mainly the one next door) to look after her at home until a few days before she died. There were many positives and blessings in this last decade of her life.

With Mum, the main rule was never to argue. No amount of reasoning ever worked, and trying to explain things usually backfired. My second rule of thumb was to distract her when things were difficult. It was so much nicer to talk about my Dad or sing along to music than to argue about when she last had a clean change of clothes. And then, when she was feeling happy and relaxed again, she would often do what I asked her to – she wanted to help me out. I was perhaps tricking her a little – but my intention was to keep her as calm and happy as possible, whilst persuading her to drink enough, and to be as clean and tidy as she would have been in the past.

After years of trial and error, I realised that I could help her more if I looked straight into her eyes and smiled a lot. This might sound strange, but it worked for both of us. And my biggest ally was to try to imagine what it would be like in her shoes. To realise that she could not see it from my point of view no matter how much I explained things – to understand that she was always going to think that she was running her own life – even though the opposite was true.

This perspective changed the way I behaved and felt – impatience and frustration often melted away. My tone of voice, body language, and the way I approached the situation probably altered for the better. When I stopped fighting, so did she – and then we usually found another way around the problem.

It also helped to be more relaxed and less perfectionist about things. There were days when it really was OK if she didn't have a proper wash or if she had more coffee and biscuits instead of her lunch.

These are the things that I found useful. My sisters found different ways around things – we had three different relationships with our mother. There is never a one-size fits all approach to caring for a relative with dementia or a brain injury. There's always going to be trial and error (and usually a lot of error!). But it is often possible to find ways around difficulties and happier ways of relating to the person.

Chapter 29: Introduction

Frances Vaughan

Jody and I started meeting for a chat and a cup of tea after her first stroke, a few months before she had the second one. We already knew each other a little, as colleagues in the university. Jody had helped me when I was setting up a research project about mindfulness and brain injury.

As soon as we began to talk about her stroke, it was clear that Jody had an unusual ability to describe her experience of the haemorrhage itself, and how she felt different afterwards. People often struggle to describe what a stroke or brain injury feels like on the inside, or to say how they have changed. Jody was aware of many of the changes she had been through, and could describe in detail what they felt like.

I was captivated by Jody's vivid descriptions and experience. We began to talk about writing a book together. Jody needed some persuasion on this – she had no idea that she was unusual. The idea that reading about her experience might help other people with a stroke or brain injury grew on us both over time. Jody would write her story, and I would add a commentary from a clinical neuropsychologist's perspective.

Despite Jody's unusual insight and ability to reflect on her experience, I did not expect her writing to be as powerful and compelling as it is. Jody's willingness to share her story, and the darker moments of her recovery, is an immense gift. I am privileged to have been part of her journey.

Clinical neuropsychologists work with individuals and families to help them make sense of their experience of a stroke or brain injury. Understanding what has happened to them can help people begin to come to terms with the losses involved. My contribution to Jody's book reflects my own understanding of her experience. It is based on Jody's writing and on the many fascinating conversations we have shared over the years.

Understanding Jody's stroke

What is a sub-arachnoid haemorrhage?

Jody became ill and collapsed very suddenly. She was later found to have had a sub-arachnoid haemorrhage. This is a kind of bleed in the brain. It is also referred to as a type of stroke.

Jody had a severe headache, nausea and projectile vomiting, blurred vision and then loss of consciousness. The pain, which is often described as a 'thunderclap headache', was intense and sudden. A stiff and painful neck and sensitivity to light are other common symptoms of a sub-arachnoid haemorrhage.

An artery that supplies blood to the back of the brain had burst. The blood was spilling out, under pressure, into the area around it. The blood escaped by flowing between two thin layers of tissue, membranes that are wrapped around the brain rather like clingfilm. These membranes are also known as the meninges – the protective layer affected by meningitis.

The sub-arachnoid space between the membranes is normally filled with a cushion of fluid that bathes and protects the brain. But when blood gets into this space (or into the ventricles, which are large fluid filled cavities inside the brain), it irritates and injures the surrounding brain tissue.

Why did Jody's artery burst like that?

The wall of her basilar artery had developed a weak spot. The weakness had created a bulge in the artery wall. The bulge looks like a balloon, and is called an aneurysm. The pressure of blood flowing through the artery eventually ruptured this bulge, and the artery bled out through the hole in the wall.

The vast majority of sub-arachnoid haemorrhages are caused by a ruptured aneurysm. Some people are born with a tendency to develop aneurysms, and this can run in families. Women are more likely to have a sub-arachnoid haemorrhage than men, and women aged between 40 and 65 are most at risk. Afro-Caribbean people have a higher risk than Europeans.

High blood pressure, smoking, alcohol and substance abuse also increase the risk of a sub-arachnoid haemorrhage. Medication to thin the blood, blood disorders and other abnormalities in the arteries can also cause bleeding inside the brain. In some cases of sub-arachnoid haemorrhage, no clear cause is identified.

Jody's hospital treatment

Jody's haemorrhage was diagnosed with a CT brain scan. CT and MRI scans can detect bleeding in the brain, strokes caused by blood clots, tumours, bruising, swelling, infection and other signs of brain injury.

Jody was moved from a local general hospital to a specialist neurological centre, and had a surgical procedure called endovascular coiling to prevent any further bleeding. This was carried out under general anaesthetic.

Three tiny metal coils were placed inside the aneurysm. The coils sealed off the aneurysm so that it could not bleed again. They were inserted into an artery in Jody's leg, and steered up through her body to the damaged artery at the base of her brain.

Jody's early medical recovery was described as relatively straightforward. She was in intensive care for a short while afterwards, and was discharged from hospital ten days after the haemorrhage.

What are the effects of a sub-arachnoid haemorrhage?

A sub-arachnoid haemorrhage is a very serious medical condition. The chances of survival are slightly better than 50:50, and the majority of people who survive have long-term difficulties.

The bleeding reduces the blood supply to areas nearby. The escaped blood can increase the pressure inside the brain, cause a dangerous swelling of the brain, cause spasm in blood vessels which can trigger another type of stroke, and cause hydrocephalus (water on the brain).

The haemorrhage often causes severe inflammation throughout the body, which can lead to other complications, including organ damage or failure. The inflammation also increases the risk of having a further stroke.

Ischaemic strokes and haemorrhages

A sub-arachnoid haemorrhage is quite a rare type of stroke. Most strokes, often called ischaemic strokes, are caused by a blood clot blocking an artery, rather than by bleeding.

Blood clots can develop in an artery in the brain and eventually block it. Or they can form somewhere else in the body and travel up to the brain in the bloodstream.

The further an artery is from the heart, the narrower it becomes. When a clot reaches a blood vessel that is too narrow for the clot to pass through, it can get stuck and block the blood flow.

A blockage stops the blood from reaching the brain cells that need it. Brain cells need a constant blood supply to survive. They begin to die at a rapid rate if they are starved of oxygen for just a few minutes.

Each area of the brain is responsible for particular actions and abilities – controlling our movement, speech, thinking and memory, for example. And so, a blockage in one particular area usually causes a specific set of difficulties – for instance, a stroke in the visual cortex at the back of the brain can cause a form of blindness.

Ischaemic strokes usually affect one particular area, usually on one side of the brain. Even a large ischaemic stroke tends to injure one or two areas in particular.

Jody's haemorrhage was described as a 'large bleed', and its effects were not limited to one particular area. The blood had spread around the outside of her brain and into the ventricles. The space under the base of the brain, where the main arteries join together to form a central loop, was described as 'entirely filled with fresh blood'. There was evidence of inflammation, of swelling at the top of her brain, and early signs of hydrocephalus.

Overall, there are two different kinds of bleeds. In Jody's case, the blood was forced into the space around the outside of the brain. More often, an artery inside the brain bleeds directly into the surrounding tissue. This is called an intracerebral haemorrhage. In both cases, the escaped blood injures the brain around it.

Confusing terms: haemorrhage, stroke and brain injury

Although Jody's haemorrhage was a type of stroke, it can also be described as a brain injury. Jody had been attending a brain injury service, and, like most people, did not realise at first that a stroke is also a type of brain injury. These differences and labels can be very confusing.

The term 'brain injury' is often used when someone has injured their head in a fall or a road accident. When a head injury is severe enough to damage the brain inside the skull, or results in a lengthy loss of consciousness, it is called a traumatic brain injury (or TBI). Strokes and other types of injury are sometimes referred to as non-traumatic brain injury or acquired brain injury (ABI).

Although a TBI is caused by an external injury to the head and a stroke is caused by internal bleeding or a blockage in the blood supply, they both disrupt the normal workings of the brain. The whole brain becomes less efficient, and different areas cannot communicate with each other as they did before.

Jody's sub-arachnoid haemorrhage will be referred to here as both a 'stroke' and a 'brain injury'. Her stroke was unusual, but it was still a stroke, and Jody had much in common with other stroke survivors. 'Brain injury' is more general, but it reminds us that the effects of a stroke overlap with the effects of a severe head injury.

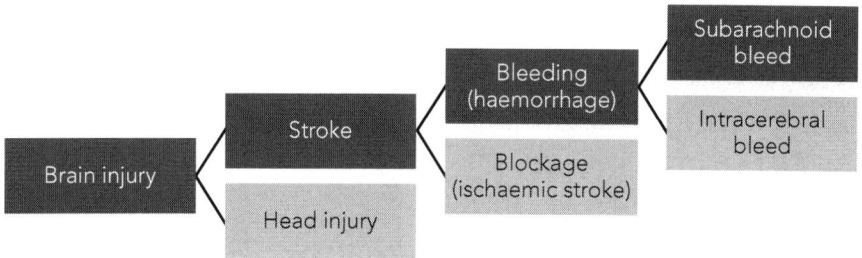

This diagram describes the main types of brain injury, strokes and bleeds. The dark grey boxes apply to Jody.

Other types of brain injury happen when the blood supply of oxygen to the brain is reduced, e.g. by drowning or suffocation. Brain infections such as encephalitis and meningitis can also injure the brain.

What are the main effects of a brain injury?

A stroke or brain injury of any kind usually causes a number of core difficulties. These include memory and concentration problems, being slowed down, tiredness, poor sleep, headache and dizziness, and emotional changes such as irritability, tearfulness and anxiety.

Other symptoms depend more on the kind of injury it is, and on which areas of the brain have been affected. For example, a traumatic brain injury (TBI) often causes significant memory problems, and alters the way the person behaves.

After a TBI, other changes will depend on which part of the head was struck in the accident. This is because different parts of the brain are responsible for different physical and mental capabilities – how we move, perceive the world, think, remember, feel and behave.

The effects of an ischaemic stroke will depend on the size of the stroke, which side of the brain was affected, which areas become disconnected by the stroke and which blood vessel was involved.

Speech and language is controlled in the left side of the brain (in right handed people), and a stroke there can cause problems with understanding language, speaking, reading and writing. Injuries involving the front of the brain tend to affect movement, memory, planning and organisation, or personality and behaviour.

How did Jody's stroke affect her?
Jody had many of the core difficulties mentioned above, as well as others that are less common. She could not remember some of her past. People's faces, and places she knew well, looked different. Her mind often felt blank, and she felt that the haemorrhage changed her as a person.

Jody's second stroke
Eleven months after Jody's sub-arachnoid haemorrhage, she had another different type of bleed in her brain. This was a subdural haemorrhage, which usually involves bleeding from a vein. The blood leaks out slowly rather than surges under pressure, and so it is often less of an emergency. Jody was taken to the same regional neurological hospital, and was looked after until she was well enough to go home again. She did not have any surgical treatment.

A subdural haemorrhage also bleeds into a space between two of the meninges, the membranes wrapped around the brain. The blood collects between the outer membrane, the dura mater, and the arachnoid membrane below it. This space, and the blood in it, was slightly further away from the surface of the brain than it was in Jody's first haemorrhage.

A subdural bleed can be triggered by a blow to the head or an infection, or it may happen spontaneously, particularly in older people. The cause of Jody's second bleed was never identified. She collapsed, but could remember the event clearly afterwards. She was physically well enough to leave hospital within a few days.

Physical and less visible brain injury changes
Many people with a stroke have physical problems – for example, difficulty with movement and sensation in their arms and legs, or with speech and language. These can be the most obvious signs of the stroke. People with a severe head injury can also have problems with mobility and communication, although these are often less severe.

Jody's stroke caused problems with walking. She was weak on one side, and had difficulty with balance, and with co-ordinating her movements. Jody's mobility improved quite quickly within the first few weeks.

Many of the changes caused by a stroke or TBI are not physical, and are often less obvious. The person may seem to be getting better physically, but other, less visible problems, such as changes in concentration, memory, mood and personality, may not be improving in the same way. This can be all the more difficult for the person and their family when other people are not aware of the less visible difficulties.

Some changes are not only less visible, they are also more difficult to understand and to cope with. It is often easier to feel sympathy and to offer help for physical problems than it is when someone loses their temper every day.

The rest of this section describes some of the less visible changes that often develop after a stroke or brain injury. These include changes in memory, emotion and behaviour, and fatigue.

The effects of a brain injury on memory

Traumatic brain injury (TBI)

People are often knocked out or lose consciousness when they have a serious head injury. If the brain injury is severe enough, they may not come round for several days, weeks or even months. The coma is followed by a period of confusion and disorientation. The person may not recognise people they know well, or know where they are, or what year, month or day it is.

This confusion is called post-traumatic amnesia or PTA. It can last for several weeks, depending on how serious the injury is. Although they have been awake, the person may not remember anything that has happened since they regained consciousness. New memories cannot be created until this stage is coming to an end. The person will not remember who they saw yesterday or what they said.

Even after the post-traumatic amnesia has passed, the person may not remember things that happened just before the injury, or in the days and weeks leading up to it. Missing memories will start to come back, one by one, and the person will gradually remember things that happened nearer the time of the brain injury. They are unlikely to remember the incident itself.

A TBI is very likely to affect areas at the front of the brain that are closely involved in memory and behaviour.

Why does a TBI affect the front of the brain?

An injury to the front of the brain tends to occur when the body and brain are moving fast and then stop very suddenly, e.g. in a fall or in a car accident. Softer organs, including the brain, don't stop as quickly as the rest of the body, and this can cause internal injuries. The whole of the brain is shaken around inside the skull, and the brain itself is stretched, bruised and torn inside.

Injury to the front of the brain is very common because the front of the skull is narrower than the back. Rapid stopping or deceleration tends to push the moving brain forwards, squeezing it into the narrower space at the front. The brain is also torn and bruised as it collides with sharp ridges of bone inside the front of the skull.

Even if the person falls and hits the back of their head, they may still have an injury at the front of the brain. The force of the impact at the back pushes the brain forwards, injuring the front in the same way.

Memory changes after a TBI

Overall then, injury to the front of the brain is very common in TBI, and this is likely to interfere with forming new memories and with remembering old ones. A TBI also affects attention, and this affects memory too.

Difficulties with memory can improve gradually for several years after a TBI, but some problems never resolve completely. The person is likely to forget what has happened recently, and what they were planning to do. They may need reminders and prompts at regular intervals. Learning tends to be slower and more information is forgotten. These problems are generally worse for more severely injured people.

Memory changes after a stroke

Memory problems are very common after a stroke, and most people have some difficulty with remembering things. The exact effect of a stroke on memory will depend on which areas and which side of the brain have been injured and how large the stroke is. If a major artery is involved, the effects will be more widespread and severe than if a smaller artery is involved. Overall, the bigger the stroke, the more likely the person is to have problems with their memory.

If the area of the brain closest to the ears is injured on both sides, the person may have very severe memory problems. If there is injury on one side only, they may have more difficulty remembering things that people have said, or things they have seen. An injury towards the front of the brain can affect the ability to search for information stored in memory, and can cause difficulty with 'finding' the right words.

No two strokes or brain injuries are the same – and the effect on memory will vary as much as the injuries themselves.

Changes in emotion, personality and behaviour after a brain injury

The brain governs our emotions and behaviour, and so when the brain is injured, emotions and behaviour can change too. The person may experience different emotions, or express their feelings differently. They may behave so differently that they seem to have become a different person.

These changes can range from something mild and subtle that comes and goes, to behaviour that is outwardly very different. No matter how subtle they are, personality changes can have devastating effects on close relationships.

How does a injury at the front of the brain affect behaviour?
The ability to control emotions and behaviour is often affected by an injury to the front of the brain. Unfortunately, injury to the front is very common – it can be caused by a traumatic brain injury (TBI) or by a stroke (a blockage or bleed).

An injury to the area above the eyes tends to cause personality change, and behaviour that is impulsive or inappropriate. The person may not be able to stop themselves doing something, often the wrong thing. They may not be able to understand what other people's behaviour means, or understand another person's point of view, or respond sympathetically.

An injury to the area in the middle of the front of the brain tends to affect motivation. People with an injury here may lose their drive and energy, and their ability to be spontaneous. They may sit quietly, with no interest or desire to take part.

What do these changes look like?
The loss of motivation can be one of the most challenging difficulties after a brain injury. Someone with no enthusiasm or drive to get things done can be hard to persuade out of their chair. The change could be mistaken for depression, but depression has different causes and needs to be approached differently.

Reduced motivation can also look like laziness. It may be tempting to think that the person is opting out deliberately. They may say that they are going to do something, but cannot put the plan into action – they can 'talk the talk, but not walk the walk'. The same person may speak less and not express the same emotions as before.

An injury to the front of the brain can affect self-control and willpower, patience and tolerance. The person may seem self-centred, with no sympathy or concern for other people. They may be tactless or inappropriate, and not at all like the person they were before.

The injury can affect a person's conscience and ability to take responsibility for their own actions. They may seem to be stubborn and inflexible, or be angry and aggressive. These changes can seem almost childlike in nature, and are beyond the person's control.

Injury to deeper parts of the brain can cause difficulties with the control of emotions. Emotions may be exaggerated – the person may cry or be extremely happy, or switch between the two. These emotions may be out of sync with other people's feelings. The person might become louder and much more outgoing. People who were previously quite anxious and responsible may become relaxed and carefree.

More subtle changes

Changes in behaviour can also be more subtle. For example, the person may have a different sense of humour, a new tendency to be outgoing or very open and honest, or new preferences for places, people and even food.

Subtle changes in emotion and behaviour can be difficult for someone outside the family to pinpoint. People's personalities are all so different, it can be difficult to know whether someone has really changed since their injury, or whether they were always this way. But for family members, subtle changes can be as distressing as more obvious changes.

Caring for a relative with a stroke or brain injury can be very stressful. Caregivers often benefit from help and support from other people who understand this stress. Information and education about stroke and brain injury, and especially about how their relative has been affected, can help enormously. The impact of changes in emotion and behaviour on family relationships will be discussed later on.

> ### It's Lenny but more so
> A young man had a serious head injury in a climbing accident. His face and forehead hit the rock face in the middle of the fall and he fractured the skull bone above one of his eyes. He also broke a leg.
>
> Lenny showed clear signs of concussion, and possibly a brain injury. During his first week in hospital, he was restless, talkative and skipped quickly from one subject to another. He couldn't stop himself interrupting other people, and sometimes made blunt or critical comments without considering their effect on others.
>
> His uncle said at the time – 'Well, it's Lenny, but more so'. Lenny had always been talkative, quick-witted and sometimes a bit outspoken, and the temporary changes after the accident were an exaggeration of his natural personality. Someone who didn't know Lenny might have thought his head injury was more serious than it turned out to be.

This uncertainty crops up in more severe brain injuries too. Unless you know the person beforehand, it can be difficult to know how much they have changed. Families are usually in the best position to make this judgment.

However, even this rule of thumb does not always work. An older woman with a severe injury to the front of her brain behaved in such a difficult way that it could only have been related to her injury. And yet, people who knew her before the accident often dismissed her outbursts, her inappropriate and often risky behaviour and her cavalier attitude, because she had always been lively, outgoing and outspoken.

Her injury had exaggerated her previously flamboyant personality. Unfortunately, the problems it caused were not always taken seriously – by her friends, and even by her family and their GP.

Changes in personality, and obvious or unpleasant changes in behaviour, are usually very difficult to absorb into family life. Changes in emotion and behaviour cause more stress for families than any of the physical effects of a brain injury.

How did Jody change?

Jody was more open and friendly with strangers than she had been. She found a new sense of connection with people, 'that deep sense of knowing them' (Chapter 9), and a loosening of the usual social constraints.

Some people become quiet or withdrawn after a brain injury, while others become more chatty or affectionate than they were. This type of personality change was part of how Jody felt different in herself.

Jody talked more than she had before, and often noticed that she didn't know when to stop. She was more impulsive than she had been, and she went through a stage where she felt less concern and empathy for other people.

Jody felt strongly connected to her family, but less connected to others she had known before her stroke. Jody couldn't 'read' other people's intentions and emotions as well as before, but she knew that the changes in her personality and behaviour were difficult for other people too.

Fatigue after a brain injury

Jody had been run over by a steamroller

When Jody came out of surgery, she felt as though she had been run over by a steamroller. Every part of her body was intensely painful, she was weak and could barely move. Jody commented that it was strange to have such strong symptoms in her body as a result of a brain haemorrhage.

General pain and weakness are very common after a stroke, especially early on. It might be caused by general inflammation, which is the body trying to protect itself from the effects of the stroke. All serious brain injuries and strokes trigger general inflammation, and it is particularly common and severe after a sub-arachnoid haemorrhage.

Jody also had muscle weakness, especially in her right leg. Many people with a stroke have some weakness on one side of their body. It might be in the leg or the arm, or sometimes the whole side of the body. Muscles can also become tight and stiff (and painful) after a stroke, or they might go the other way and become floppy.

Jody also felt completely exhausted. This was an extreme form of tiredness that Jody had not experienced before. Exhaustion is extremely common after a stroke, both straight away and, in some cases, for a long time afterwards. Fatigue can be very severe even when the stroke or brain injury is relatively mild. It involves mental exhaustion as well as physical fatigue, and the person may feel confused or suddenly at a standstill because of it. Fatigue can make other problems worse than they would be otherwise – for example, concentration and memory are often affected by tiredness.

This tiredness and lack of energy, called post-stroke fatigue, improves gradually, but may still be a problem for months or even years. If sleep is also affected by the brain injury, as it often is, this can make the fatigue worse. However, even people who sleep well can also have severe fatigue.

The effects of the fatigue

Long-lasting fatigue is another challenging problem caused by a brain injury. Tiredness and lack of stamina limit how much people can do. People often feel frustrated, low in mood, irritable and impatient because they are so tired. Managing fatigue by planning around it can often improve mood and pain, as well as the tiredness.

Planning for fatigue

People with fatigue can run out of steam very suddenly. It may not depend on how much they have done, or how long they kept going for. It can be hard to predict when it will happen. However, learning to recognise the triggers and the early warning signs can help people to manage fatigue. The person may always be exhausted after an hour in a crowded room. They may have slurred speech or become unsteady on their feet as the tiredness kicks in. Other people may recognise the warning signs before the person with the injury does.

The section below looks at some simple strategies that might help you to manage fatigue.

Things that can help with fatigue

Spreading activity out across the day and across the week can be very helpful. Planning ahead can help to avoid doing too much, exhaustion, and the need for a long period of recovery. A little and often is better than boom and bust.

Starting to do things before you are tired. Resting before you start to do something again.

Thinking about how long you are busy for rather than how much you have done. Decide to work in the garden for an hour - rather than setting out to weed the whole flowerbed.

Other people may not understand the problem and may try to persuade you to do more than you can manage. Helping others to understand the fatigue and the difficulties it can cause can reduce misunderstanding and tension.

Fighting with fatigue

It can be difficult to accept that you cannot do as much as you used to. It is not unusual to want to fight the fatigue, to battle on regardless, until you drop. This is can be part of a accepting the brain injury as a whole, and coming to terms with its effects.

It can be particularly hard to avoid exhaustion when you are having a good day. You might feel as though you could go on forever. But doing too much will probably have exactly the same effect as it did the last time, and it may be better to stop before you feel that you need to.

You may be worried about being misunderstood – that others will think you are lazy or selfish because you do less than they do. It may feel embarrassing or shameful. Giving clear information and explanations can help, as well as being clear about how much you can do, and sticking to it.

Coping with fatigue

Resting, perhaps before and after a busy period is important. Make sure you have eaten enough. Having enough blood sugar is important for stamina.

You may feel embarrassed or guilty about the need to rest, that you 'should' be doing more, or that you should be back to 'normal', when this is impossible for now.

It is important that relatives and friends understand that fatigue after a stroke or brain injury is not the same as ordinary tiredness. The fatigue does not always depend on how active you have been, or on how severe the injury was.

The understanding and support of relatives and friends may help you to manage your fatigue. Knowing that the brain injury causes fatigue may help them to encourage you to rest and pace yourself.

Fatigue can bring up a lot of distress and other concerns about the brain injury. This is entirely natural. It is hard to predict how long the fatigue will last for and it is a difficult problem to cope with, especially when other things are getting better. Talking about it with people who have similar problems can help, or asking for professional support in managing the fatigue.

Jody spent a lot of time resting in the first weeks after her stroke – it was essential for her early recovery. Unfortunately, though, many people continue to be very tired despite resting properly and pacing themselves.

There is currently no medical treatment or cure for the fatigue. It can be managed to some extent, by taking things slowly, and resting between activities. Working around the exhaustion is usually better than trying to fight it.

Cognitive changes after a stroke or brain injury

Jody vividly describes how her stroke affected her memory and her ability to concentrate and to think clearly. When someone asked her one more question, all the oranges fell out of the orange bowl. The tsunami of her mind swept away her memories and threw them into a heap far away. These are powerful descriptions of Jody's internal experience in the aftermath of her stroke. They speak for themselves.

At the same time, neuroscientists and clinicians working in rehabilitation have a growing understanding of how the brain works and what happens when things go wrong. Some of this background might also be helpful here – to better understand what Jody experienced and how a stroke can affect our abilities.

The next four chapters describe the difficulties that Jody had from a neuropsychology perspective. Neuropsychologists often use the word 'cognitive' to describe the brain processes that govern our intellectual or mental abilities. Cognitive processes are the invisible workings of the brain that allow us to make sense of the world – to speak, read and write, to concentrate and remember, to solve problems and to make decisions.

Cognitive Changes After Jody's Stroke

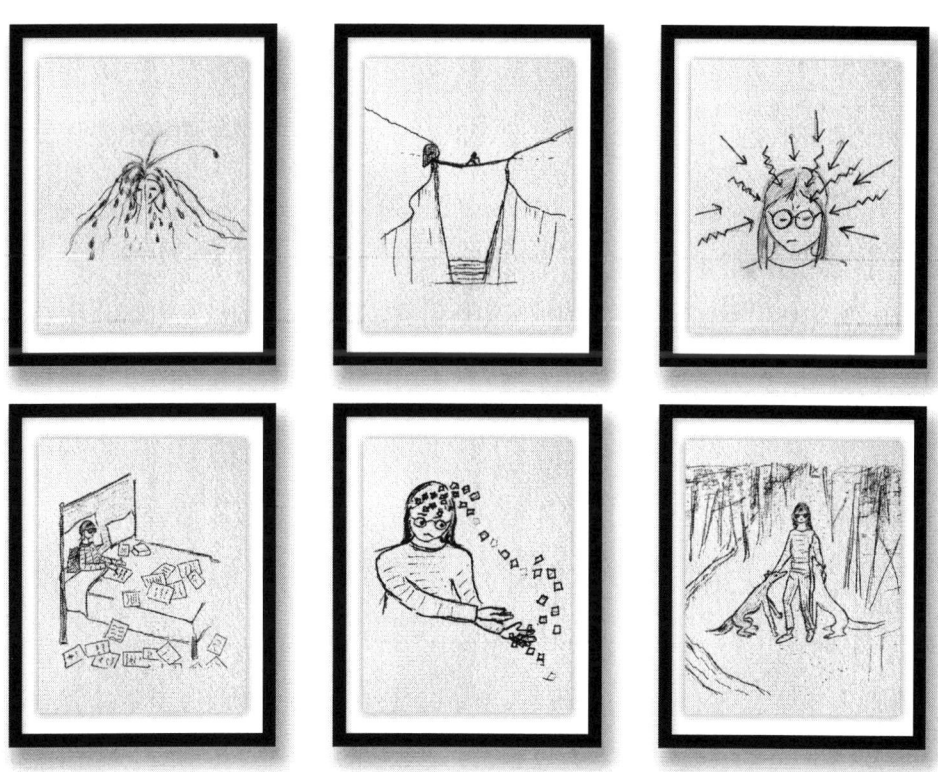

Chapter 30: Attention

Problems with attention might be a good place to start this exploration of Jody's cognitive difficulties. But why should attention be the best place to begin?

First of all, attention forms the cornerstone of all the cognitive processes. Attention is like the foundation of a pyramid, creating a stable platform for perception, memory, language, thinking and planning processes.

Attention is an essential part of everything we do; it allows us to concentrate for long enough to finish a task. It allows us to focus on that task while ignoring everything else that might distract us. The ability to control our attention is crucial to the smooth running of our lives, as Jody discovered when controlling her attention became very difficult.

Second, attention is critically important in mindfulness and meditation. Jon Kabat-Zinn's well-known definition reminds us that 'Mindfulness means *paying attention* in a particular way: on purpose, in the present moment and non-judgementally'. Beginning to meditate again after her stroke made Jody realise that she could not pay attention in this way for long.

Finally, problems with attention are extremely common after any stroke or head injury, even a relatively mild one. It is very easy to underestimate attentional problems, which are not always immediately obvious, and to mistake attentional problems for something else. For example, problems with attention can cause forgetfulness or confusion.

Jody's attention was severely affected by her stroke. This was a double whammy – not only did Jody's problems with attention affect her everyday life, they made it impossible for Jody to sit and practice mindfulness, an essential part of her life before the stroke.

What is attention?

At first sight, the answer to this question might seem obvious. 'Pay attention!' We all know what that means. We use attention when we concentrate, and we know what concentration feels like. We are very tuned into attention, especially in other people, but it is hard to imagine what attention actually is.

When we concentrate, we need to keep our attention going. If it's noisy, we also have to stop ourselves being distracted. If we're doing something new or difficult, we need total concentration, and we cannot think about anything else.

And so, attention is not just one thing that the brain does – it involves a whole team of brain processes, all of them tuned into what we are doing and trying to achieve. Some basic processes keep us alert, or monitor our surroundings for signs of danger. Others manage the flow of information around the brain, and move attention backwards and forwards between tasks.

Attention processes are carried out in specialised neural networks that are spread across the brain. These circuits work together and communicate with networks that supervise other activities.

Part of this system is like a filter, a bridge between the outside world and our brain. It decides which parts of our surroundings and body we need to be aware of, and which we can safely ignore. It identifies things that need further processing, and helps us to ignore the less important stuff. This system evolved to keep us alive – so that we could find enough food, and see our predators in time to escape them.

Attention controls the flow of information from one cognitive process to another. It affects how fast information is processed, how much information is allowed through and which information is given priority. Its job is to filter, focus and then process the important bits. A brain injury tends to affect all of these functions.

The human brain can only deal with a certain amount of information at a time. We all have a limited amount of 'head space'. A healthy brain works around this problem by being fast and efficient. Unfortunately, an injured brain not only has less space, it also operates more slowly and cannot filter out unimportant material. People with a brain injury often feel overwhelmed by information and cannot deal with it all at once.

A slower brain and sensory flooding

After her stroke, Jody's brain was slowed down and could not handle as much information at once. She had a sense of not being able to 'keep up' with the world, and of being overwhelmed by the speed of things: 'other people seemed to move in a faster, louder world – seemed to speak so quickly – I couldn't follow them. What I often heard was a shouted jumble of words' (Chapter 2).

Jody's brain had also lost an important defence mechanism – a filter that holds some sensations at bay. We are constantly bombarded by sensations that we don't need to respond to, and so they are filtered out or processed unconsciously. We are simply not aware of them.

We often don't hear background sounds. We don't usually feel our feet touching the floor, or see the colour of the table we are sitting at. We don't have to deliberately ignore these sensations; they are filtered out before they reach our awareness.

Imagine being woken up in the middle of the night and finding yourself in a fairground. Surrounded on every side by loud music, bright coloured lights, flashing and chasing around the outside of every ride. Amusement machines making loud noises, some squawking, shrieking, dinging – a huge wall of loud noise. Add to that the sickly-sweet smell of candy floss, a burger grill, hot dogs and frying onions. It sounds like a nightmare – we would all want to hide under the duvet.

For Jody, ordinary things such as crossing a busy road or going to a shopping centre were as overwhelming as a fairground. Unfortunately, she had nowhere to hide. Places that were crowded and busy, brightly lit and full of strong smells seemed chaotic; she could not make sense of them or cope with them.

The filter was not working properly, and Jody's senses were flooded and overwhelmed. For her, there was no background noise, only noise. Perfume and aftershave smelled unbearable. The volume had been turned up on all of Jody's senses after the stroke, making her feel more sensitive to everything.

Because Jody's filter didn't work properly anymore, she often felt overwhelmed and could 'crash' like an overloaded computer. Her ability to think and make decisions disappeared.

A healthy brain cannot deal with every sensation, which is why the filter evolved in the first place. So, Jody's brain had an impossible task – it was already slowed down, but had all the unimportant stuff to deal with as well.

Sensory flooding can be triggered by sights and sounds that are too 'busy' – too colourful or bright or loud. It can block out a conversation, so that the person is effectively hearing impaired. For some people, loud noise, such as loud music or traffic noise, can even be experienced as physical pain.

New and unfamiliar places can be more overwhelming than familiar ones; dealing with new information takes more energy and is tiring. This can produce a vicious circle – people feel more overwhelmed when they are tired.

Sensory flooding is extremely stressful – it creates anxiety, fear and, at times, panic. The brain misunderstands the overstimulation and sees it as a danger signal. The body goes into a state of red alert, ready to fight for survival or run away. This is helpful when we are in real physical danger, but it does not help with sensory overload, as the stress response interferes with thinking and reasoning. Furthermore, long term stress is bad for our physical and mental health, and so being severely overwhelmed on a regular basis can cause additional stress-related problems.

For Jody, her sensory overload was at its worst immediately after her stroke and has improved over time. Jody has also learned to cope with it, by sitting and breathing, finding quieter places to go and avoiding certain types of situations. She discovered which places she could tolerate and made changes that helped, e.g. softening the lighting in her office.

As Jody's control over her attention improved, she was able to ignore some of the more troublesome invasions from her senses. This takes effort and repeated practice, but it works for some people and can reduce stress.

Jody's image of her cup was helpful too. 'I imagined myself being able to climb into such a space and just sit there – supported by the curved sides of the cup – all the loud sounds and flashing objects seen out of the corner of my eyes would be calmed – somewhere to rest for a while within the chaos of my head' (Chapter 9).

Complex forms of attention

As we have seen, the brain usually filters out unimportant sensations automatically, without our conscious awareness. More complex forms of attention involve greater awareness, and more conscious mental control.

We know when we are concentrating well and when we are distracted, and we can make an effort to concentrate better. We can control our attention by directing it towards things that are important to us at that moment. We can switch attention backwards and forwards between things, which allows us to multi-task. We can even attend to two things at once – listening to the radio while driving is a classic example. This ability to control attention allows us to survive in a complex, demanding world.

Concentration

Jody had difficulty with concentration in some situations. She could not do formal mindfulness practices for several months after her stroke, and she described her attention as 'all over the place'.

However, she could concentrate on physical activities such as painting, drawing, tapestry and crochet for long periods of time. Indeed, Jody became immersed in these, and concentrated on them for much longer than she did before the stroke.

If things are done slowly and at the person's own speed, and if there are few distractions, people with a brain injury can often concentrate well.

Ignoring distractions

Being able to focus on one important thing while ignoring something less important lies at the heart of what we mean by attention. This 'selective attention' is often described as a spotlight. The 'light' moves around, often following the movement of our eyes, focusing on the things we need to be aware of.

We are not blind to things outside of the spotlight, but we are more intensely aware of things that are lit by it. We can change the size of the spotlight. We can focus on a very small area, or we can widen the focus and take in more information more slowly.

The idea is that we point the spotlight at the things we need to know about. Less important things outside the spotlight beam can still distract us, and 'pull' the spotlight over to them. Everything around us competes for our attention all the time.

Fortunately, we have some special attention mechanisms that help us to ignore distractions. They dampen down our response to things we can safely ignore, and speed up our response to important things. However, these mechanisms are also quite fragile, and are less efficient after a brain injury. Unimportant things are no longer ignored automatically – instead they cause distraction and information overload.

Mindfulness and attention

When Jody began to meditate again she listened to recordings made by other mindfulness teachers. The recordings guide the listener through each mindfulness practice, step by step. The instructions are extremely helpful for most people, especially when they are new to mindfulness.

Jody found it difficult to follow these practices, even though she knew them well. She could not keep her attention on her breath or her body, at least not for long. Focusing on sensations that were not very tangible may have made this more difficult. Perhaps Jody could concentrate on her tapestry for longer because the physical objects and movement involved drew and held her attention better.

Moving the focus of her attention along in a sequence was particularly difficult. Jody did better if she focused on just one thing.

One of the first things that people experience when they begin to meditate is that their attention wanders, often very quickly. This is natural and normal; it's what our minds do. We start to think about something else, or we are distracted by something we hear, and that triggers another train of thought.

The mindfulness teacher tells the listener to expect this, inviting them to bring their attention back to the breath or to the body, without judging themselves. The teacher's guidance can be very helpful in this respect – it provides an anchor for attention, bringing it back to the breath when the mind has wandered.

Jody was easily distracted by things around her. Jody may have been so distracted that she could not bring her attention back to the meditation. Jody's fatigue also reduced her ability to meditate. Focusing and re-focusing attention on something, especially something intangible, requires a lot of mental energy. This would have been more challenging when Jody was already tired.

Jody learned to meditate again despite these difficulties. She continued to use the recordings, but switched to short, three minute or ten minute practices. She built it up gradually, often repeating the same short practice two or three times in one session. If she had tried to do a different, 30 minute practice, her attention would probably have collapsed again. Adapting to something new or different took time and energy.

Jody noticed that many of the practices she listened to had 'too many words' for her. She found the guidance distracting, but at the same time she needed an external anchor for her attention, to help her maintain her focus.

In contrast, Jody had the most difficulty with a practice known as 'choiceless awareness'. This has no specific instructions, and no particular focus for attention. She found it difficult to stay focused on anything at all.

Through determined and dedicated practice, Jody regained greater control of her attention and was able to meditate without the recordings. Eventually, Jody went back to teaching mindfulness again.

Jody's spotlight of attention

Despite being easily distracted, Jody spent a lot of time in a very focused state of attention, where the beam of the spotlight was narrow and intense. As we have seen, this happened when Jody returned to her crafts and hobbies, and began to play games again. She spent a long time immersed in them.

Jody's long and intense focus on things, and the way she found it difficult to move from one activity to another, was almost certainly related to her stroke. Jody told me that she often felt 'stuck' in things, and that it was difficult to tear herself away. It was often an external event, such as a knock at the door, that would bring her back to the world and prompt her to stop what she was doing.

This tendency to be immersed in something often goes hand in hand with distractibility. It may seem strange that the same person can be distracted at times, and intensely focused, almost stuck, at others. In fact, this is quite common, because they both involve the voluntary control of attention. Jody could be distracted and 'all over the place', but she could also be stuck.

'Going wide'

Jody could also have a very wide focus of attention – so wide, in fact, that she found it frightening to begin with. 'Going wide' was an awareness of the space around her that expanded until it included an awareness of the whole world and outer space.

It began with Jody's awareness of her body, of her body in the room, in a building, in a town, a country, and so on, out into space and the stars. Jody described the wide as a 'huge, zoney place' that she could have lost herself in; she was often caught up in the wide when she watched the sea and the sky through her bedroom window.

Jody had a sense of floating out in space or on the sea, aware of everything in the universe, but less in touch with her own solid form. Jody commented that there was 'not much identity in space'. Jody was sometimes afraid of getting lost in it, and of being unable to get back.

When the wide focus felt unsafe, Jody imagined her cup as a place to sit and feel safe. She had a 'body sense of the image' – feeling the cup around her contained Jody's attention and stopped her going too wide.

At first, Jody's focus changed from narrow to wide, and back again, on its own. Jody practiced changing the width of her attention during meditation and gradually achieved greater control. She brought her attention back to her body and then gradually widened her focus again, to sounds, then to her thoughts, and further out into the world and beyond.

The wide focus was like the 'choiceless awareness' mindfulness practice that Jody had found difficult at first: it had no specific focus, and there was nothing to contain Jody's wide attention.

Later in her recovery, Jody used a wide focus of attention to help her to cope with headaches, fatigue and overwhelming sensations. She found that 'widening' around these difficulties was more helpful than turning towards or focusing on them, which her mindfulness practice would normally have encouraged her to do. This allowed her to carry on with things, rather than stopping or lying down. She could stay with the headache, fatigue and overwhelming sensations, but they were just a part of her wider awareness, rather than its focus.

Jody used a wide focus to cope with difficult situations, such as being stuck in a tunnel on the London Underground. She held an image of the train and the people around her, the different levels of the Underground above them, going up to the street, and then up to the sky and the stars above London. This allowed Jody to feel very calm in a situation that was difficult for her.

Jill Bolte Taylor's 'Stroke of Insight'

There are parallels between Jody's wide focus of attention and Jill Bolte Taylor's experience of a haemorrhage in the left side of her brain. Jill and Jody both had a sense of vast space around themselves, and a strong connection with present moment experience, rather than with thoughts.

In her book *My Stroke of Insight*, Dr Jill Bolte Taylor, who studies neuroanatomy, describes her experience in terms of the difference between right and left brain functions. Her perception of herself and the world changed dramatically during the haemorrhage. When the left side of her brain closed down during the bleed, Jill had an intense meditation-like experience. She explained that this was created by her non-verbal right hemisphere, which was still functioning.

Jill's capacity for logical thought dissolved, came back and went again. The familiar stream of thoughts, plans and comments was either silenced or not making sense. With the left side of her brain temporarily out of action, Jill experienced a world that was timeless, silent, peaceful and spacious. She experienced herself as pure energy, connected to the consciousness of all other humans. It felt like nirvana. She was absorbed in sensation and the wonder of an interconnected universe.

Jody had little sense of time passing in the early weeks after her stroke. 'Everything seemed to slip away, so that there was only this moment' (Chapter 4). She also experienced a vast sense of space in 'the wide': 'I sometimes felt the walls and the window dissolve between me and the sea… I almost felt that I was out there, as much on the sea as on my bed' (Chapter 7).

We know that the right side of the brain becomes more active when people learn to meditate. At the same time, meditation reduces brain activity on the left side, in areas linked to anxiety and to our sense of self. Jody had noticed that her mind's inner voice had quietened since her stroke, and that she was less caught up in the planning, remembering, worrying and regretting that used to occupy her mind. It was as though Jody's stroke had also induced a more meditative state of consciousness generally, especially in the early weeks.

Jill's experiences were relatively short-lived and dramatic. Jody's were less intense but longer lasting. Nevertheless, the similarity of their experience –

of moment by moment awareness, of spaciousness and separation from the physical world and a quieter inner voice – seem to be linked to meditation-like states of consciousness and to the areas of the brain activated by meditation.

Later in her recovery, when Jody could use her verbal, thinking brain more effectively, she adopted her wide focus of attention as a coping strategy in difficult moments.

Switching attention backwards and forwards

Jody thought that she had stayed out in 'the wide' for hours at a time. She may have been stuck in that wide focus of attention, just as she was often caught up in a very narrow focus.

Later, when Jody was working again, her attention was often captured by a particular topic of conversation or teaching point. She sometimes had difficulty moving on to the next topic without a reminder or prompt.

Many people with a stroke, brain injury or other neurological condition have 'sticky' attention, and cannot move their attention around flexibly. As we shall see in a later section, this can be associated with other forms of inflexible thinking and behaviour.

Doing two things at once

People often attend to two things at once – talking and preparing a meal at the same time, for example. Dividing our attention might slow us down, and increase the chances of making a mistake, but this will depend on how similar the two tasks are, and how automatically we can do them.

Most experienced drivers can listen to the news on the radio while driving on familiar roads. But if the route is unfamiliar and very busy, the same driver may need to devote all their attention to the road until the traffic eases off. They might not hear the radio any more, or they may switch it off.

Jody could rarely divide her attention after the stroke. Even when driving was easier again, she could not cope with the radio or music at the same time. 'So I just drove' (Chapter 10).

Jody could not talk while making tea for a long time. As we have seen, Jody could not make tea automatically, and needed to give it her full attention. A conversation would distract her, and steal some of that attention – she might lose track of what she was doing, miss something out or stop making the tea altogether.

Holding things in mind

Conversation while making tea was a problem for Jody partly because it interfered with her ability to hold things in mind. Holding plans and ideas in mind involves attention as well as memory processes. The information we are going to need next is identified and pulled out of memory, and then held in mind until the job is done. When we no longer need to hold it in mind, we can let it go and move on.

Under normal circumstances, this continuous process of choosing and holding information happens automatically, in the background, usually without thought or effort. We can hold information about four or five things at once – essential for multi-tasking. But if this information – about what we are doing now, what we are planning to do next, what someone just said about tomorrow – literally slips from our mind, as it did from Jody's, we lose track of ourselves and where we were, and become disoriented.

Jody often had difficulty with holding her ideas and plans in mind. This was one of her most debilitating problems: 'And my head would simply empty – no memory of what I was doing – where I was… I could feel the space where the information had been before my attention was taken away from it' (Chapter 15). It seems that Jody had to pay conscious attention to anything that she needed to hold on to. Once her attention had gone, the information went too.

Overall, Jody did not have 'as much' attention as she needed after her stroke. She needed more but had less. The second difficulty was that she could not control her attention as she had done before. She could not easily move her attention, divide her attention or use it to ignore distractions and hold information in mind.

The attention manager

The attention system described so far cannot work efficiently on its own. It doesn't know what it is aiming for. It needs to be supervised and controlled by a more senior group of brain systems, which we might call the executive control centre or the manager.

The manager is aware of our purpose in life at any given moment, and is driven by our goals and how important each one is. Attention is tuned into these goals and concerns. What is important, and what can be ignored depends on what we are aiming for.

The manager works out how alert you need to be. It decides whether it is safe to divide your attention between two things, or whether you need to stay focused. It runs some familiar tasks on 'autopilot', allowing more attention to go to something more demanding. It decides what can be ignored and what needs to be in the spotlight. It switches our attention between tasks at the right time.

Attention can be captured by a sudden event such as a loud noise or an emergency siren, but the manager returns your attention to the task in hand when the disturbance has passed.

The manager is a complex system of neural circuits spread across the outer layers of the brain, mainly towards the front. These circuits communicate with other brain networks, which in turn control other abilities, such as memory, perception, language, thinking and planning.

Things that can help with attention difficulties

When a task needs your full attention, making a plan can be helpful - decide where and when to do it.

Choose a calm quiet place, where there will be no interruptions.

Drawing the curtains, wearing headphones, switching off the phone and the TV, and putting a 'do not disturb' notice on the door – keeping distractions away.

Doing difficult things when you feel most alert and refreshed, perhaps in the morning or after a rest. Concentrating is tiring anyway, so you need to be at your best. If the task is long and boring rather than difficult, breaking it up into short sections to do one at a time, can help.

Discussing concentration difficulties with family or friends, particularly the people who need to leave you alone for a while.

Doing one thing at a time. Going backwards and forwards between tasks can make them both more difficult.

Taking a break if you feel tired and your concentration is lapsing. A change of scene and a rest can make all the difference.

Avoiding deadlines and time pressure if at all possible. Feeling anxious about what you are doing will make your concentration worse.

For families and friends

Almost everyone with a brain injury has difficulty with attention and concentration. Most people are also slower to take in and to respond to new information. These changes are a direct result of the injury, and the person has no control over them. They may need support with doing things in everyday life, such as dealing with official letters or making decisions.

You may need to remind the person to go to a quiet space to do anything they need to concentrate on. You may need to help them to organise this.

Remind them to do only one thing at a time, so that they avoid feeling overwhelmed and distressed.

If you are telling the injured person about something new, giving them the information they need without hurrying. Give them enough time to keep up with you, and to take the information on board.

Try to organise the day so that there is space between things, to allow for some rest and relaxation before the next thing.

Chapter 31: Memory

As we have seen, people with a brain injury almost always have problems with memory. Some people can remember things they knew before the injury, but cannot easily learn new information. People often forget what has happened or has been said, or what they planned to do later.

Finding things in memory

Jody's image of the haemorrhage as a torrent of blood, ripping up everything in its path and hurling it about, conveyed how difficult it was for her to remember things after the stroke. The landscape of her mind had changed, and she could not recall things she had known for many years. Some memories were lost forever; others were swept away and buried somewhere, hard to find.

Jody's description of 'a jumbled heap' (Chapter 2) also reflects this difficulty. It is hard to find anything in a jumbled heap. A heap of socks needs to be sorted into pairs, and organised into individual piles, before we can easily find our own socks.

Memory is much the same – finding something quickly and easily depends on our memories being sorted and stored in a logical way. Sifting through them one by one would take too much time and energy, and even then we may not find what we're looking for.

Information stored in memory is linked together in complex and highly organised networks of information – like a three dimensional spider's web. Everything in this network could, in theory, be linked to everything else stored there. One of the biggest advantages of this is that you can search for things in more than one way.

Imagine looking for a lost wallet. You check the rooms you've been in recently. You look through the clothes you've been wearing. You search the car. You call the train station and go back to the supermarket. You search all the places you've been to since you last used it, but you don't waste energy going anywhere else. You develop a line of attack, a strategy, based on what you have done recently – looking in the most likely places first. This is how memory works when it's working well. A search based on strategy is very different to a random search.

Looking for the wallet by retracing your steps makes total sense. But if you hadn't used the wallet for a year, your search would be very different. There would be no point in going back to the supermarket.

Searching our memory is the same. There is usually more than one way to find something. Our brain changes the way it searches, depending on what we're looking for and why.

Think about your favourite mug. If someone asked you to, you could describe its colour, its weight, what it feels like to drink from, the glaze and pattern on the outside, where you bought it, how much it cost, how long you've had it for, when you use it and where you keep it. It might only be an ordinary mug, but you know a lot about it, and you can bring that information to mind in an instant.

You could have brought the same mug to mind in a different way. Suppose your favourite mug is blue and it was given to you last Christmas. If you were asked to describe all the blue things in your kitchen, you would eventually have 'found' the same mug. Or if you were asked about gifts you have been given at Christmas, or about your belongings that are quite new. The stored memory of your mug contains all these features; the mug is coded as blue, as a Christmas present and as something new.

When we can't remember a person's name, we often try a different way of finding it. We think about the letter it might begin with, or about the names of the person's relatives. We can search our memory in many different ways, based on different features and from different starting points. Without this, remembering anything would feel like looking for a needle in a haystack, as it often did for Jody.

Although Jody felt as though the stroke had swept her memories away, they had not really moved. It was more likely that Jody's brain had lost the ability to search her memories efficiently, and so couldn't find things easily or quickly.

When Jody and I discussed this idea of not knowing how or where to find her memories, it seemed to fit with her sense of having 'no known pathway' through her memory any more (Chapter 2). Jody had to find her way around and learn to make links between things again.

People with memory problems can often recognise something they have seen or heard before, but cannot bring it to mind for themselves. The information is stored somewhere in memory, but they cannot find it. If a person with memory problems is given prompts and things to choose between – was it this or that? – they may be able to access more of their memory.

Memory problems may be attention problems

If we walk into our home and have several people talking to us at once, we may not remember where we put our keys when we came in. We can only remember things if we pay attention to them as they happen. And as we have seen, a brain injury usually causes difficulties with attention.

Some people with memory problems do surprisingly well on memory tests when they have the chance to pay attention properly. Their 'memory problems' may be more of an attention problem. Attention can often be improved more easily than memory – and so it is important to know what is causing the difficulty.

Memories are stored in different areas of the brain

The brain stores different types of information in separate memory networks. For example, the way you remember a big sporting event will depend on whether you heard it on the radio or saw it on the TV. Some things are stored in memory for words, or in a separate memory for things we have seen – faces, pictures, landscapes or maps.

A brain injury often affects one type of memory more than others. Jody could remember pictures and images more easily than words.

The importance of knowing where things were

The brain has separate stores for information about where things are and the information we use to find our way around. Jody had particular difficulty with both types of memory for places.

Jody forgot where things were at home. Over time, Jody learned to keep some things in their own special place, which helped. However, Jody's main strategy was to keep everything out, on the desk or on tables, so that she could see them.

Piles of paper were clearly labelled, and once Jody looked at the label on the top of the pile, she would remember what was in the pile. The labels gave her a 'way in' to recalling what was there, and she could reconnect with what she was doing.

It was important that the piles of paper were not moved. Otherwise, Jody couldn't remember what was in the piles, even with the labels to look at. Her work plans and domestic paperwork were 'anchored' to those piles and, particularly, to the place she kept them in. Looking at them in that place unlocked the memory of her plan and how far she had progressed. They were an essential part of the scaffolding Jody created to help her manage things.

A few years ago, Jody and I gave a talk at a conference in a hotel. We needed a quiet place to chat beforehand, and I went see Jody in her hotel room. Jody was upset when I arrived because the cleaner had (with the best of intentions) tidied up all of her belongings and piles of paper, and Jody had no idea where anything was. We slowly rearranged everything and eventually Jody could find her way around them again.

Jody could not change her jumbled memory, but by keeping the piles of paper in the same place, she had built an external memory system to rely on instead.

Getting lost

Jody could not keep track of where she was in an unfamiliar place or building. She couldn't find her way out because she had no memory of where she had come from. The example of Jody getting lost in the ladies' showed how frightening this could be (Chapter 6).

Jody could not remember new driving routes. She had little sense of direction, and in unfamiliar territory she did not know where she was in relation to where she was going. Jody had to rely on a satnav to drive outside of her home patch.

Places are an important part of what we remember. We often know where we were when things happened in the world and in our own lives – many of us remember where we were when the news of the attacks of 11 September 2001 first broke. Having a clear sense of where we are allows us to remember things in more detail, and not knowing where we are interferes with this.

Memory for actions and doing things

We have another separate memory store for how we do things and the movements involved. Some actions – such as riding a bike or walking – are hard to describe in words. This kind of memory stores instructions and skills that your body knows the feeling of and how to do. People with severe memory problems, who cannot recall their recent life at all, often have this 'muscle memory' and can do things they learned many years ago.

In the early days of Jody's recovery, she could not remember how to do everyday tasks, such as brushing her teeth. Jody had to learn them for a second time. Although she knew what to do once she had been shown, she needed help to get started and everything felt strange and difficult at first. Re-learning required Jody's full attention and effort.

Jody had particular difficulty with the c-ordination of movements and sequences of movement. Jody continues to have difficulty doing things in sequence, which is not unusual after a stroke. Jody's early attempts to do things in sequence depended on having everything she needed laid out in front of her.

Everything she needed to make tea had to be out on the tea tray, and the sequence broke down if just one item was missing. If the milk had been moved, Jody did not know what to do next. It stopped her in her tracks, and she couldn't carry on without it.

When everything was there, tea making flowed smoothly from one stage to the next. Each item on the tray prompted Jody to take the next step. She didn't have to remember anything, or search for things. Jody could practise something that she could not yet manage entirely on her own.

These skills improved with practice. But for a long time, Jody found that taking everything out and putting it in the right place before she began to do something was very helpful.

Some memories last longer than others

Memories are stored in different networks for different lengths of time. We can hold small amounts of information, such as a telephone number, for a short time. Other memories are stored more permanently, and some can last a lifetime. The following sections describes the different kinds of memory store we have, and some of the difficulties that Jody had with each one.

Working memory and holding things in mind

Jody's difficulty with holding things in mind was discussed briefly in the chapter about attention. Holding things in mind was one of Jody's biggest problems – things slipped away from her mind when she stopped paying attention to them.

We often hold thoughts and plans in mind for a short while. We need to know what we are going to do later today, or what we just went upstairs for. This ability depends on attention and memory operating together, in a system called working memory.

Working memory can store small amounts of information for a short time. We might repeat a phone number to ourselves until we can write it down. When we stop paying attention to it, the number fades quickly and is gone.

We can hold bigger chunks of information for longer than this, although not permanently. An example of this is the mental 'to do' list that we keep ticking over in the back of our mind – the kind of information that Jody lost when her memory slipped.

This store helps us to keep track of our progress with the things we need to do soon. You might have put the kettle on earlier, and need to go back and make the coffee. You might have to remember a plan – to meet outside the cinema just after 6, but if it's raining, to meet in the café across the road. The details of the plan may be forgotten soon after the cinema trip, unless something memorable happens on the night. Things are ticked off the list and forgotten when we don't need them anymore.

This temporary store is not always strong enough to stop other ideas and distractions breaking in and replacing items on the list. Keeping distractions and interference at bay is particularly difficult for people with a brain injury.

Jody's difficulty with holding things in mind

Jody made sense of this difficulty using the orange bowl metaphor. In the beginning, Jody's orange bowl could only hold one orange. Gradually, Jody's ability to process information improved, and she could keep two oranges in the bowl – as long as no one brought her a third one. The extra orange distracted Jody, and interfered with the oranges already in the bowl. The first two were forgotten and she could not hold on to the new one either.

Jody learned to cope with this problem by keeping all of her work tasks separate and doing only one thing at a time. This allowed her to work without putting too many oranges in the bowl at once.

Following a conversation presented the same problem: 'if I let my attention stray, I know it will all roll away and I will not remember any of it' (Chapter 6). Jody could stop it rolling away sometimes, but more often, the effort made things worse and the idea disappeared anyway. These memory slips affected every part of her life. It was like losing the thread of a conversation – and with it, Jody's sense of continuity and purpose.

Looking back on her experience, she commented on how much information we try to hold in memory: 'what we have done – memories – what we are going to do next – what that will lead to in the long term… we hold so much' (Chapter 16).

Memory for recent events

We have a separate memory store for things that have happened recently – a film we saw last week, what we ate for dinner yesterday or what people have said in recent conversations.

Jody often forgot recent experiences, particularly recent conversations. Jody often needed a reminder of what we had spoken about and agreed to do. During the conversation, Jody thought that she would remember it all. She did not expect to forget the conversation when she stopped thinking about it.

Jody made notes to remind herself. Writing things down often helps people to remember things later, because we pay attention to them as we write. However, this did not seem to work for Jody, who also forgot to look at the notes later, as she had intended to.

Knowledge and our life history

Everything we have learned and know is held in another separate memory store: the history and geography we were taught at school, the names of plants and animals, the names of streets in our town, our family tree, the Highway Code and the meaning of all the words we know.

Jody had lost a lot of this longstanding knowledge, especially information she had used in her work. She also had word-finding difficulties, which is very common after a brain injury. This added to her sense of having a blank mind.

We have another separate memory store for the events of our lives. These may be childhood memories, or memories of more recent times. Jody could not remember important parts of her early life and some parts of her adult life. She could find small 'pockets of memory amid the rubble' (Chapter 3) but the whole landscape of her mind was never fully rebuilt. Trying to recall things was a huge effort, particularly in the beginning.

As Jody's ability to search her memory slowly improved, some of her missing knowledge and life story came back to her. These memories had always been stored in her brain, but Jody had not been able to find them.

Remembering to remember

Remembering to do something in the future involves another type of memory. This ability is an important part of our busy lives. Some things have to be saved for later, e.g. we can only call to make a doctor's appointment during office hours. We must remember to call when the surgery has opened, and before it closes again.

If it happens regularly, forgetting to do things later can cause a lot of difficulty in everyday life. It happens to everyone from time to time, which is why we rely on diaries, calendars and mobile phones as much as we do. However, people with a brain injury often have great difficulty with this.

'Remembering to remember' is a distinct type of memory. It is not linked to remembering new information or things from the past. Problems with this often go hand in hand with planning and organisation difficulties. The smooth running of our lives depends on remembering to follow things through and sticking to the plan. These memory problems often disrupt the plan, and cause further difficulty and frustration.

In the first weeks after her stroke, Jody often forgot to do things she meant to do. These were often ordinary but important things, such as making a drink and taking her tablets. Often, Jody would only 'remember' to do this when she felt thirsty or realised that her headache was getting worse.

Out of sight, out of mind

We usually know when something we need is missing, and we can usually work out what it is. We know what should be there. Jody's experience after her stroke was quite different. As Jody put it herself: 'If it was in front of me, it was there. If it wasn't, then it didn't exist' (Chapter 2). When the milk was missing from the tea tray, Jody didn't know what was missing or what to do next. The milk was out of sight, and out of mind.

This out of sight, out of mind problem is difficult to understand. Surely everyone would realise that the milk should be there? At this early stage in Jody's recovery, she could only respond to things that she could see. Other things did not exist and it was hard for Jody to work out else she might need.

Most of the time we can only see a few of our belongings, but we know that the others are there. We can think about them and we know where they are. Jody could not do this. Anything that was put away in a cupboard or drawer 'ceased to exist – it would never come out again' (Chapter 16).

Jody had the same difficulty with people, especially with people she did not know well. It took a few months for new people to become real to her, to build a picture of them in her mind and to develop an idea of their identity.

Eventually, Jody managed this out of sight, out of mind problem by organising her surroundings differently. She labelled things, gave away belongings and made sure that everything she really needed was kept in sight.

Jody commented that this was like a stage of development that babies go through (Chapter 2). An older baby will understand that a toy still exists even when it is hidden under a blanket. Older babies lift the blanket and find the toy. Younger babies behave as though the toy does not exist, as Jody did when something was out of sight. Being able to remember things that we can't see is an important human capacity, and losing it causes difficulty, as Jody's experience illustrates.

Jody still needs important things to be in view. Like many of us, she prefers to print her writing out rather than read it from a computer screen. However, the paper also makes the writing feel more real and permanent. This is a mild form of Jody's out of sight, out of mind experience.

Filling in the memory gaps

In the early stages, Jody's memory problems made her mind feel blank and empty. This was difficult emotionally as well as practically.

Jody was embarrassed when she discovered that she repeated herself and that the story wasn't always the same. People with memory problems often repeat themselves, and 'fill in' the things they don't remember with something that sounds quite plausible. Relatives and friends may think that they are making it up, but that is not what the person intends or experiences.

Things that helped and things that hindered

Whether Jody can remember something or not also depends on how she is in other ways: how tired she is, how well she can concentrate, how interested she is in something and whether or not she is feeling anxious or upset.

These factors affect everyone's memory, but after a brain injury they are even more important. Jody's fatigue and difficulties with attention often made her memory problems worse.

Jody often stopped trying to remember and took some time out instead. It was important to stop, sit, have a drink, do a mindfulness practice and see whether things came back to her on their own. Often things did come back, most often when Jody stopped trying to grasp them.

New learning and a better landscape

In Chapter 4, Jody wrote: 'Here I was unable to remember anything much, never mind what day it was, what happened yesterday, what I might have said to someone on the phone this morning, what was on the radio half an hour ago.' But then, to her delight, Jody found that she could learn poems from her new book by heart. It was a remarkable contrast.

The poems brought together some powerful influences that helped her to learn them. Jody loved poetry, and was motivated to improve her memory and learn again. Poems often have a strong emotional resonance, and a rhythm that make them more memorable. Jody may have also remembered the poem's 'footprint', the visual pattern the verses made on the page.

Jody later read a novel for the first time since her stroke. It was also poetic and lyrical, and the rhythmic writing may have made the book easier to read and hold in mind.

Jody found that she could remember pictures more easily than words. She could remember an idea better if she associated it with an image in her mind. Imagining two things together is a well-known strategy for improving memory. As in other situations, Jody excelled at designing her own rehabilitation programme.

Jody re-discovered old skills, such as dancing the waltz and sewing a tapestry. She noticed that these had stayed with her and came back fairly easily, with none of the problems she had with more recent learning and memory.

Many of Jody's memory problems improved over time. Her most persistent difficulties involved holding things in mind, searching her memory for knowledge and words, finding her way around, and remembering where things were. These improved gradually and Jody's approach to remembering became more organised. She developed strategies that reduced the impact of some of these memory problems.

The following information is for people with memory difficulties and the people who support them. Family members may need to remind and prompt the person to use their memory aids.

> ## Things that can help with memory
> Understanding the person's memory problems more clearly, perhaps through a memory assessment. Knowing which aspects of the person's memory are most affected can point towards the best ways to support them with it.
>
> ### Mobile phones and other technology
> Electronic devices, especially smart phones, can be used in different ways to give prompts and reminders.
>
> Creating reminders using electronic calendars, voice recordings and alarms on mobile phones. A note about what to do when the alarm goes off can be added when you set the reminder up.
>
> Taking pictures of things you plan to use later. For example, a picture of your wheelie bin to remind you to put it out later.
>
> Using just one or two of these methods, and developing strong habits in the way you use them.
>
> It can be a challenge to keep track of the reminders, and to remember why you set them. If you make voice recordings or take pictures, you will need to remember to go back to them later.
>
> Using automatic bank payments so that you don't have to remember to make each one.
>
> continued >

Traditional memory aids

Traditional reminders and prompts can be just as useful as electronic devices. These might help with memory problems:

Keeping a pad of paper by the phone to make a note of any messages.

Using a diary or a calendar (although not both). Having one central place for all the information you need, and keeping it where you will see it all the time.

Using a diary to make a note of appointments and social events in the future. You might want to make a note of things you have done to refer back to later.

Using a diary with large pages to make a daily plan, a shopping list, as well as a record of what you have done each day.

Being more organised can help too:

Having one place to keep the things that usually go missing – keys, phone, glasses, wallet etc. Putting these back in the same place every time.

Having a checklist of things to take with you when you go out.

Making a plan for each day, and a list of things you need to do.

Ticking things off when you have done them – you are less likely to miss things out.

Using post-it notes for important reminders and putting them where you will see them. Or using highlighter pens in the diary or calendar.

Throwing away letters or papers you don't need any more. They will cause confusion if you leave them lying around.

Putting tablets in a pill organiser box marked with the days of the week, and keeping it where you will see it.

Labelling things in cupboards and drawers to keep them organised and easy to find.

Setting an alarm on a kitchen timer as a reminder to do something there later.

Routines and helpful habits

Having a daily routine and doing things at the same time of day every day. You will spend less time and energy looking for things and working out what to do next once the new habit has become routine.

Making a checklist for your new routine until it is established.

Going to a quiet place with no distractions to do something that will tax your memory.

Doing one thing at a time.

Checking your calendar or diary every night so that you know what is happening the next day.

Memory strategies

Paying close attention to something you will need to remember later.

Making an image of it in your mind. If you need to buy some raspberries and some washing powder, think of your car or shopping bag filled with raspberries and soap bubbles. If you need to phone the plumber and buy some dog food, imagine your dog chasing the plumber down the road. The sillier it is, the easier it is to remember.

Writing things down and reading them aloud sometimes helps to make the memory stronger.

continued >

Repeating the thing that you want to remember, over and over. For example, the name of someone you met recently. Repeating it again after a while, to build up a stronger memory.

Breaking numbers or words into groups of three. Chunks of three are easier to remember than a list. You can repeat them to yourself in a more rhythmic way.

Breaking tasks down to make each step as simple as possible, rather than trying to remember too much. Keeping things simple and organised takes the weight off your memory.

Making the best of your memory

Some parts of your memory may be better than others. Try to use the better parts as much as possible. Jody tried to remember things in pictures rather than words.

Reconnect with skills you had before the brain injury, especially things you enjoyed. Your memory for them may be better than you think once you get going.

If you are stuck and can't remember a word or what you were going to do, it may be best to leave it for a while. It may come back to you suddenly and more easily if you don't try to force it.

When you come back to it, ask yourself questions – what letter did the word begin with? This can be a way into your memory. Retracing your steps might remind you of what you were going to do.

If you have an 'out of sight, out of mind' problem, make sure you can see the things you will need. For your family – if you need to discuss something that is out of sight, having physical objects, such as a letter or a photo, clearly visible might make the situation more 'real' for the person.

Your memory will freeze up more if you are anxious, frustrated or worked up. Making a deliberate decision to stop and relax can help.

Chapter 32: Planning and Organisation

Being busy in our lives means that we have a purpose – something that we're trying to achieve. It might be to leave the house in the next ten minutes, or to be promoted in the next five years. Whatever the goal is, we know how we are aiming to get there, the steps we will need to take along the way. We know how much progress we have made. We may need to multi-task, to switch from one job to another as we work towards the goal.

Planning and organising are highly skilled complex abilities that take years of practice – and years of brain development – to achieve. Even so, many people are so practised in running a home or doing a job that this ability to juggle tasks and manage time can feel like second nature. When we are healthy, these abilities feel strong and robust. In reality, they are very fragile, especially after a brain injury.

Jody's planning and organisation difficulties

When Jody first came home from hospital, the idea of managing her medication, shopping and meals was completely bewildering. She could not work out what needed to be done, or form an intention to do things. Having someone there to prompt Jody and to keep reminding her what to do was really helpful at this stage. Jody tried to 'see back, back into then to know what I needed to do now. And that didn't work. And now I gave up to that' (Chapter 4).

For someone with a brain injury, working out what is needed, making a plan, breaking it down into smaller tasks, remembering to do them and to do them in the right order, can be extremely difficult. The person may not be able to keep track of their progress or know what to do if something goes wrong.

These difficulties are a very common direct consequence of a serious brain injury. People often need a lot of support to get back into a routine. For Jody, planning and organisation were more difficult because she was easily distracted and could not hold her plan in mind. These difficulties had a huge impact on her life for many months.

The executive control centre

Planning and organising abilities are controlled by complex networks of brain cells located towards the front of the brain. These networks form part of the executive control centre, or manager, described earlier.

This manager of the brain leads the brain's activity. Just as a factory manager makes sure that everything comes together to create the finished product, and the conductor of an orchestra keeps the musicians in time and controls the volume of each section, the manager co-ordinates the activity of the whole brain. It is devoted to keeping us on track in our lives at work and at home.

The manager and the automatic pilot

Not only does the manager work out what we need to do, it also decides how much conscious attention we need to do it. If we are driving along 'on autopilot' and there are flashing blue lights up ahead, the manager will immediately take over from the autopilot. We slow down, and pay a lot more attention to our driving and the road.

The manager allows the autopilot to run familiar routines quietly in the background, and steps in with new instructions only when there is a problem. The manager is particularly important in new or dangerous situations where the autopilot does not know what to do.

Nothing was automatic for Jody for some time after her stroke. She had to think about what she was doing all of the time. Jody's autopilot was not working properly, and without this to fall back on, she did most things as if learning them for the first time. At this stage Jody's attention and mental energy were still very limited, and so everything was very tiring.

What else does the brain manager do?

The manager looks after all aspects of our complex human behaviour. It supervises and co-ordinates the mental tools we need for being busy – thinking and reasoning, solving problems, planning, organising, making decisions and judgements, thinking ahead and being flexible. These mental tools, known as the executive functions, are complex control processes in themselves.

The manager monitors our behaviour and our progress. It decides whether we should give up or keep going. It helps us to recognise when we make mistakes and to find a different way forward. It decides when we should start an activity, how long we should keep going for and when we should stop. People with executive function problems often have difficulty with starting things, or cannot keep going, or may not be able to stop.

The manager is also responsible for our motivation and enthusiasm for life, and for the skills we use in our relationships with people – for our ability to reflect on our experience, use willpower and restraint, follow rules, show sympathy and kindness and understand another person's point of view. It is the source of invention and creativity. It allows us to achieve our goals in life.

What executive difficulties did Jody have?

In the first few weeks and months, Jody could not use strategies or solve problems. She could not search under things or look inside them. Putting things together in a sequence was particularly challenging; it was easy to miss something out, or to do things in the wrong order. She could not create her own plan of action, and she relied on external prompts and cues. As we saw earlier, Jody could not make tea unless everything was laid out for her.

Jody also had trouble with making decisions and choices. The orange bowl idea was a helpful way to understand this – if Jody had more than two options, she would lose sight of them all and the decision was impossible.

Jody needed things to stay in the same place. Moving things stopped her in her tracks. Jody's brain did not have the flexibility or the 'headspace' to deal with the change. Changes mean more information to deal with and more decisions. Keeping things the same was much less demanding.

Jody often forgot what she was planning to do next. If a plan involved several steps, she could only think about one at a time. It was impossible for Jody to look ahead, to think about what she would be doing later, without losing track of what she was doing now. Jody's first train journey to Liverpool was a very clear illustration of this. Being unable to look ahead made organisation much more difficult.

Multi-tasking has been impossible for Jody since her stroke. She could not hold plans in mind, and she could not switch backwards and forwards between them. Jody's mantra of 'one thing at a time' was exactly right (Chapter 11).

Jody's relatively mild executive difficulties were made worse by her attention and memory problems. Being organised, thinking things through and making decisions were more difficult because she was distracted or could not remember what she was doing. Indeed, Jody's underlying ability to plan, structure and organise things recovered fairly quickly, and from then on, these difficulties were less severe than her attention and memory problems.

Regular routines and structure

People with executive difficulties cope better in an organised environment. A regular routine and having 'a place for everything and everything in its place' can be very helpful.

However, many people with executive difficulties cannot create this kind of structure for themselves. Being given prompts and instructions that break a task down into steps can makes things more doable. Without this kind of support, life for people with executive difficulties can become overwhelmingly chaotic.

In the early months, Jody's mindfulness practice, activities and games stimulated her brain and helped her to retrain her attention. They also gave her a sense of purpose, and without them she did not know what to do. Later, as Jody's recovery continued, she realised that she needed to develop more of a routine.

The way that Jody recognised this for herself was a sign that her thinking brain and her ability to organise herself were returning. Her decision to have a new puppy to care for and plan her life around was both a positive step forward and a sign of recovery.

Why did everything have to stay the same?

Jody's planning and organisation abilities were not flexible. Jody could work through a plan as long as nothing changed. If something changed, it was hard for her to create a new plan. If there was a problem on the road, Jody could not plan a new route in her head. Having to change route could be enough to cause her brain to crash.

Through the creation of strong habits and routines, Jody's tasks became more automatic and less exhausting. Although this helped her to manage her life, Jody could not be spontaneous as she had been before her stroke. She had a regular routine, going on the same walks with her dog and shopping in the same places. Unplanned trips were usually out of the question.

The familiarity of routine and habitual activities made them easier, and there was very little room for manoeuvre with this.

Moving to a different perspective

Jody's early tendency to become absorbed and stuck in something seemed to go hand in hand with other changes in her mental flexibility, e.g. the need for things to stay the same, talking more than before the injury or saying the same things. Jody often thought that she had talked too much, or that she had repeated herself; both of these can be part of getting stuck.

Being stuck can make it harder to see things in a different light. Jody could sometimes see the bigger plan but could not get a handle on the detail. She could have 'difficulty in moving from the whole vision' to the details she needed to follow the plan through (Chapter 15).

She could also get stuck in the opposite direction. 'Later I thought it was rather like watching a film – you know it is the whole film – the whole story – but can only see that one scene from it at a time – all the rest is out of sight' (Chapter 15).

How did Jody's skills improve?

Jody's ability to plan and organise herself improved gradually. When Jody went to buy the wedding tapestry set for her daughter (Chapter 4), she realised her trips out had more purpose. She had something to aim for again.

The new year after her stroke marked a turning point in the recovery of Jody's executive abilities (Chapter 7). She moved on from the games and jigsaws that had been so helpful, to real-life activities that were less structured. Jody was beginning to use reasoning and problem-solving skills, to make decisions and use strategies.

Jody learned new ways to cope with her brain injury changes. Back at work, she began to use the memory strategies described earlier – to organise paperwork into piles, to keep things in one particular place and not move them, to keep everything important in view. 'I had to be very structured' (Chapter 10).

Jody's problem-solving skills improved so much that she could use these to sidestep other difficulties. As long as Jody could remember what she was meant to be doing, was not interrupted and did one thing at a time, she could carry out complex activities. Her thinking skills had returned, and her difficulties with memory and holding things in mind did not cause quite as many problems. Almost a year after her stroke, Jody could organise her household tasks and her work materials better. She could see the bigger picture more clearly.

Despite this, keeping track of herself was still a huge challenge. Jody set reminders and alarms to help her to do things in the right order and at the right time. But these did not work for Jody, mainly because she would be distracted and start doing something else instead. Her attention problems could still get in the way of being organised.

The scaffolding built by Jody's team

Back at work, avoiding noisy and crowded places and working around what she could cope with was more difficult. Jody tried to plan things so that her brain did not crash, but this also required realistic judgements about what she could manage, and this did not come back as easily.

Jody's colleagues learned to give her the space she needed, to organise things for her and to give her prompts and reminders. They took over some of Jody's executive and memory functions. This freed Jody up to do other tasks which she was better at, to make the best use of her experience and skill. Jody commented that she was not good with the paperwork, but was comfortable in other parts of the job. These included teaching, supervision and discussion in meetings – things that involved face-to-face contact with colleagues and students.

Jody's skills coming back – a summary

Jody had difficulty with planning, the organisation of information, solving problems, keeping track of progress, making choices and decisions and thinking in an abstract and flexible way. These difficulties improved gradually over time. She worked hard to practise old skills and routines, and to find a way around her problems.

Jody's executive function abilities had been buried for a while, rather than lost. A year after her stroke, Jody could use them to get around some of her attention and memory problems.

Jody could organise and structure her work physically, which helped her to organise it mentally. Many of Jody's executive abilities worked well, as long as she could hold on to ideas for long enough to use them.

Just before the second stroke, Jody was deliberately creating a familiar structure around her work. She knew that as long as the structure stayed strong, she could cope.

Jody's second stroke

By the time Jody had her second bleed, the executive difficulties from the first stroke had improved enormously. However, there was still not much room for error. The seemingly mild second stroke brought some of these problems back and made others worse. The second wave of changes in her executive ability were harder to deal with than anyone expected.

After the second stroke, Jody could understand an overall plan, but couldn't see how it broke down into steps. She had trouble following the plans through. Work became too difficult and Jody decided to resign.

Jody's own way of doing things

Jody could not use the strategies that other people recommended. She tried to use lists to organise her shopping, but she often forgot to take the list with her, or forgot to use it in the shop.

This 'remembering to remember' problem is very common after a brain injury, and there are no easy solutions. Some people find that mobile phone reminders are helpful, but this doesn't work for everyone. Jody's solution was to sit and breathe, to accept that her memory problems would keep on happening and not blame herself.

Jody did not have the flexibility or 'headspace' to use devices and reminders to keep her on track. Mobile phone alarms, voice recordings, electronic calendars and flow diagrams were too complicated and confusing. Jody could not remember how to use them.

They also took up so much space in Jody's mind that there was no room for the information she needed to remember. People found this difficult to understand, but a paper diary and organised piles of paper were much more helpful. Jody commented that 'There isn't a better system – just the one you know.'

> ### Things that may help
> Some people's executive difficulties are more severe than others, and people need different amounts of support. However, the same advice is helpful for everyone. It is also similar to the approach used for attention and memory difficulties – many people have problems in all areas.
>
> #### Things that may help you with planning and organisation
> Using planners can help you to be more organised, and help you to remember to do things later on.
>
> A whiteboard can be useful as a general planner for appointments and social events, a shopping list and a place to write things down before you forget.
>
> You might prefer to use a diary or calendar. Whichever you use, developing the habit of putting notes and reminders in the same place and the habit of looking at them regularly can help.
>
> #### Planning and organising a task or activity
> When you have a particular job to do:
>
> Making your surroundings as calm and uncluttered as possible. Tidying up before you start.
>
> Reducing distractions as much as possible.
>
> Doing things before you are tired. Fatigue will make things more difficult.
>
> continued >

Making sure that you have enough time. Feeling under time pressure can be overwhelming.

Writing a plan for the task, a list of the steps involved and instructions for each step if needed.

Talking to yourself! It really helps to keep asking yourself questions. What are you doing now? Do I have everything I need? What else should I be doing? How much progress have I made?

Giving yourself instructions all the time. Saying things out loud will make you think clearly about what you're doing.

If you tend to be distracted or spend a long time doing nothing, set a regular alarm on a phone or timer. When the alarm goes off, ask yourself the same questions. What was I planning to do? Where am I up to?

Support that family and caregivers can give

A person with executive difficulties may need a lot of prompting and support. This can help them to make the most of their other abilities, and make the most of their rehabilitation and therapies. You may need to provide the planning and organisation that the person cannot do for themselves.

The person may need to be reminded of their difficulties, such as their memory problems. They may need to be prompted to use reminders on their phone, or their whiteboard.

The person may need help with staying on track. They may need to be prompted to do something, even if they have not forgotten about it.

Developing a routine and keeping things in the same place can be very helpful – the person will have less to remember and think about. Routines become easier and more automatic with practice.

Suggest new activities that are not too demanding. Tasks and activities are easier when they are broken down into manageable stages, with clear instructions for each step. Remove unnecessary steps and keep the instructions as straightforward as possible.

The person may have to do things one step at a time, rather than trying to do the whole task.

Avoiding time pressure, taking things slowly and having regular breaks can reduce frustration and increase the chances of success.

Use reminders and planners that are clearly visible to the person, and develop a habit of looking at them together.

When difficulties come up or the person has gone 'off plan', asking them to stop and think about what they are doing can be very helpful. Ask them to say what they were planning to do, how much they have done and what, if anything, has gone wrong.

Give positive feedback about progress and sensitive feedback about any errors. Help the person to see where they have gone wrong, if they have. Discuss the next step. Make suggestions or give reminders about this if necessary.

Chapter 33: Perception

What is perception?
Our eyes, ears and other sense organs send a constant stream of signals to the brain – and the brain's job is to makes sense of those signals. It puts them together to give us a complete 'picture' of our surroundings. Perception is this process of making sense of the world around us and where we are in it.

The brain does this smoothly and seamlessly. We are not aware of perception; it happens automatically, without any effort on our part. Perception comes together mainly in the back of the brain, in specialised networks of brain cells. Perception involves many stages of information processing, and any of these stages can be affected by a stroke or brain injury.

Visual illusions can help us to understand more about perception, especially the idea that perception happens in our brain, rather than in our eyes. When we are misled by a visual illusion, our brain has been deceived. It can be tricked into seeing something that isn't there, something that Jody experienced on many occasions.

The effects of a brain injury on perception
After a brain injury, some people cannot recognise certain types of things – everyday objects, familiar places or the faces of people they know well.

The person can see the object clearly, but their brain cannot make sense of it. The brain literally does not know what it is. This type of problem was illustrated beautifully in Oliver Sacks' book *The Man Who Mistook His Wife for a Hat*.

When faces are not recognised, the person may identify someone from their clothes or the sound of their voice instead. When my daughter was a toddler and I had just been for a drastic haircut, she didn't recognise me in the nursery playground. She said: 'I can hear my mummy's voice, but I can't see her face'. A recognition difficulty caused by a stroke or brain injury might feel very much like that. Puzzling and perhaps quite frightening.

Everything looks different now
Jody's perception of the world changed after her stroke. She had 'new eyes that can look with wonder at the world' (Chapter 1). Jody saw more detail, and more beauty, and the world was brighter and more vivid than before.

Jody found it hard to bear when her 'new eyes' perception began to fade later in her recovery.

The world also looked different. Her daughter's flat looked different. Jody's own house 'looked like the wrong house but felt like the right one' (Chapter 2). It may have looked wrong, but sounded and smelt familiar.

Familiar places looked strange and different – a nearby town and the library in Jody's village. But then Jody realised that she was remembering them as they had been, perhaps 40 years before. The strange appearance of things may have been as much about Jody's memory as it was about perception. Things did not look the way she expected them to.

Perception and memory affect each other

Memory and perception are closely related in our brains. Our memories are based on how things look, sound and smell and how they make us feel. A stranger's face, music or a fragrance can remind us in an instant of something from our past. When things did not look, sound or smell the same as they did before, Jody could not connect to her memories in the same way. This was another barrier to remembering things from the past.

Seeing movement that wasn't there

Jody could often see things moving when they were standing still. Walls and shelves seemed to lean over, as though they would fall on her. Trees and lampposts moved. The roadside seemed to waver at the side of her vision.

These movements were an illusion created in Jody's brain and caused by her stroke. Movement receptor cells were being triggered into action by mistake. They usually only work when things move in front of our eyes. Although there was no movement to see, Jody 'saw' it exactly as if it was real. Visual illusions are a helpful way to 'see' movement and other effects that are not real.

The image shown opposite ('Hold on Tight' by Gianni Sarcone) creates an illusion of up and down movement in the drops or bubbles, and the lines appear to wave and wobble. If you don't see the bubbles moving up and down on the page, have a look at a larger colour version online: https://pixels.com/featured/hold-on-tight-gianni-sarcone.html

The waterfall and the rock

Anything that moves in front of our eyes will trigger the movement receptors in the brain. Some cells are triggered by things moving upwards. Others respond to things moving down. This works perfectly most of the time, but the brain can be tricked into seeing movement that isn't there.

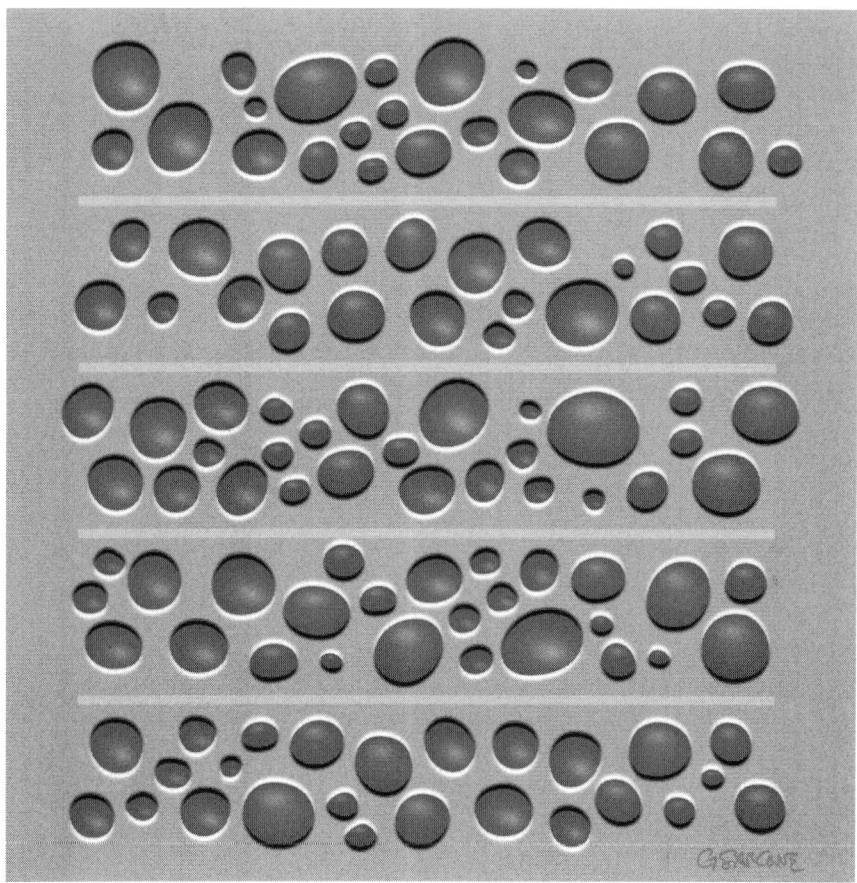

Licensed Image. Gianni Sarcone/ Pixels.com.

You can see this for yourself the next time you are by a waterfall. Stare at the waterfall for around 30 seconds without moving your eyes, and then move your eyes to a nearby rock. The rock will appear to move upwards.

Jody's brain injury may have upset the balance between her 'up' and 'down' perception. Looking up at the shelves full of toys in the superstore, or crowded stacks of books in the bookshop, may have been like looking at the waterfall and the rock. Tall shelves, high ceilings, tall trees and lampposts all seemed to trigger this illusion of downward movement.

Long enclosed spaces seemed to set off Jody's 'up' receptors at the wrong time. The road seemed to be rising up when they drove home through the tunnel. The supermarket floor seemed to be coming up towards her when Jody walked down a narrow aisle.

The car park illusion

We can all experience this kind of illusion. When we drive along a road, lampposts and houses seem to be moving past us. This is an illusion, because we are moving past them. Anything that seems to be moving past us tells our brain that we are moving.

But even this perception can be misled. If you sit in a car park or on a train in a station, and the car or train next to you begins to move backwards, you can easily feel as though you are moving forwards. You see this movement out of the corner of your eye, and your brain mistakenly works out that you are moving, rather than the train or car next to you. It can be terrifying when the car seems to be moving off on its own!

Jody often saw illusions of movement at the edge of her vision, especially when she was moving in a car. We are more likely to see false movement at the edge of our vision than in the centre. Peripheral vision has lots of gaps in it, which the brain tries to fill in. Jody's brain may have filled in these gaps with signals from her unusually sensitive movement receptors.

3D viewing

For a long time after her stroke, Jody was often overwhelmed by TV programmes and films at the cinema. Things that moved quickly triggered the perception that they were moving towards her in 3D. It could also make Jody feel that she was moving, and that she might fall over. Again, receptors in Jody's brain were being triggered at the wrong time to create an illusion of movement.

An overloaded brain

Jody was more likely to see illusions of movement when her senses were overwhelmed or she was very tired. She saw the walls falling in on her when she was in busy, noisy places, or surrounded by high, crowded shelves. Her senses were already overloaded, and her brain was more likely to make mistakes. If she was sitting quietly at home, the walls were usually still.

However, other perceptual changes that Jody experienced cannot be explained by sensory overload.

Face recognition

Jody did not recognise her own face immediately after her stroke, and she continues to be surprised by her face in the mirror. Friends' faces also look different, as though they have changed in some way. Jody may have remembered a 'younger version' of her own face and other faces she had known for a long time. Or there may have been a fundamental change in the way she perceives faces. This is not at all unusual after a stroke affecting specific areas of the brain.

Jody did not always understand the emotions expressed in other people's faces. There are special brain networks involved in perceiving faces, recognising familiar faces and understanding facial expressions. Jody's stroke may have affected all of these face areas.

Jody did not recognise acquaintances from her village. Jody could sometimes get to know them again by staying and talking. By the end of the conversation, she often had a sense of them and of her relationship with them. Jody might not have recognised their face, but their voice and the things they talked about were often familiar.

More about getting lost

We saw earlier that Jody could get lost in unfamiliar buildings because she could not remember where she had come from. On top of this, she could not make sense of the space around her and where she was in it. This disorientation in space made her memory problems worse.

Jody could not work out where she was, e.g. which side of the building she was in or where she was in a unfamiliar town. She could not use distinctive features to find her way around – to understand where she was in relation to where she wanted to go. She could not recognise that passing the bottom of the stairs on her left side meant that she was walking towards the front of the building.

Jody no longer had a good sense of direction and could not build a 'mental map' of the space she was in. She literally did not know where she was and could not keep track of where she had come from and was going to.

People with this kind of spatial disorientation often have difficulty recognising even familiar landmarks and using them to work out where they are. They may have to stop and ask for directions many times before they can find their way. Some people with this difficulty also have problems with face recognition.

Scrambled sensations

Jody noticed that her senses could be muddled up, that one type of sensation could be experienced as another. For example, 'sometimes with loud music, I seemed to be able to see the sound' (Chapter 7). This happened for a long time after her stroke, and it still happens when she is very tired.

Experiencing one sensation as another, called synaesthesia, is quite usual for some people, although Jody had not experienced it before. Instead of perceiving sensations separately – so that sounds are only heard, and pictures are only seen – perception in the brain is altered so that the senses merge or are more closely connected.

Jody often felt there were slabs moving in her brain, particularly when her memory slipped. She also had a sensation of cold water running inside her head. This is not unusual, especially after a subarachnoid haemorrhage. Jody experienced these unusual sensations against a background of shooting pains and almost constant headache, for which she took pain relief throughout her recovery.

Time perception

What is time perception?
Time perception is our awareness of time passing and our ability to keep track of time. It is based on attention and memory, and holding things in mind. We have no sense organs for time in the way that we have eyes and ears for sight and sound – there are no time detectors.

Time is perceived using a large network of brain cells that stretches from the back of the brain to the front. The network contains a kind of biological clock that pulses or ticks like a real clock, and keeps time in the brain. Some neurological conditions are known to affect time perception.

What do we use time perception for?
Time perception gives us a sense of time. The past, the present and the future are a part of everything we think about. Our memories and our plans are shaped and organised around time. We travel backwards and forwards in time, all of the time.

We use it to remember our lives more clearly, and to make sense of the past. Our memories are anchored to a point in time. A sense of time grounds us – without it, we can become confused and disoriented.

We keep track of the time constantly. We know roughly how long we have been waiting for, or how long something will take to do. If we are asked to call back in ten minutes, we will know when to do it, give or take a few minutes. We can estimate how many weeks have passed since something happened – a holiday, or the last time we spoke to a friend.

The experience of time
We can lose track of time, or we can be watching the clock. Time goes faster when we are enjoying ourselves, or under time pressure, or are very busy. If we are bored or fed up, time can pass very slowly. We can lose track of time when we are absorbed in something, as Jody was with her tapestry.

Keeping track of time takes attention. If we are immersed in something, our brain may be too busy to track the time as well. People may lose track of time after a brain injury, because they have less attention available to do this.

Being in natural surroundings – such as a wood or a beach – and feelings of awe and wonder can create a sense that time has slowed down.

Jody's time perception

Jody had very little awareness of time passing. She often did not know what the time was, or how long she had been doing something for. Jody had no structure to her day at first. There was almost nothing she had to do at a particular time. There was only now.

As Jody recovered, her sense of time improved but did not fully return to its previous state. Jody's difficulties with time were quite severe, in keeping with her attention and memory difficulties.

When Jody was out and about again, her sense of time caused difficulty. She went to the local shop when it had already closed. She was often late for meetings and appointments because travelling took longer than she expected.

Having no sense of time and being easily distracted created a vicious cycle. Jody was more easily distracted because she had no sense of time. Her sense of time was worse when she was absorbed in the thing that had distracted her. Jody asked colleagues to time things for her, to tell her when a meeting should be coming to an end. But even then, Jody could lose track again and carry on the discussion.

Mindful awareness and time

In the early days of her recovery, Jody was often in a state of 'flow', immersed in the sea and sky, or absorbed in an activity. She was quite unaware of time passing.

She instinctively adopted a mindful awareness of the present moment from the beginning of her recovery. This was enormously helpful in many ways, but it added to her sense of timelessness. Focused activity and meditation both steered Jody towards a more timeless state.

Being absorbed in meditation and repetitive activities suited Jody's needs and her abilities during her early recovery. However, it was difficult for her to move back into a more timetabled and hurried world.

How did time affect Jody's memory?

Having little sense of time did not improve Jody's memory problems. Awareness of time helps us to lay down stronger memories. Time is wrapped up in the memory when we create it, and this can help us to recall it later. A sense of time gives us a fuller, stronger connection with the memory.

It was harder for Jody to remember to do something later because of her sense of time. The brain circuits involved in time perception and remembering to do something later overlap with each other and work together.

> **Things that can help with time perception**
>
> Increasing your awareness of time may help you to manage your time better.
>
> Having a clock or an egg timer in a very prominent position can make the passing of time more obvious.
>
> Timers, alarms and time management apps are built into many electronic devices. Anything that prompts you to think about the time, what you are doing now and whether you should move on to something else can be helpful. Alarms can be set up to go off regularly (eg every hour) or randomly.
>
> If you have difficulty keeping track of time, observing things as they happen around you might help. Noticing the arrival of the postman or newspaper, hearing children going home from school, or the lunchtime news programme on the TV might help you to become more aware of the time.
>
> Focusing on an event, rather than a particular time, might help you to remember to do something later. For example, you might remember to switch the oven on when the children come home from school – rather than aiming to do it at 4pm.

The Hum

The Hum began at a difficult time in Jody's journey. Her capacity to deal with new sounds was already low. Her sensitivity to sound had been turned up by the first haemorrhage, and loud situations were still difficult to cope with. She was also easily distracted by unimportant sounds and the Hum grabbed her attention.

Jody was also less resilient than before; her mood was low and she was more anxious generally. This made the Hum more difficult to cope with.

After the initial shock of a background sound like the Hum, people often begin to adapt to it and gradually notice it less. Unfortunately, it was the opposite for Jody, who perceived the Hum to be growing louder, stronger and more insistent. It was always there, and it was everywhere.

The Hum drowned out some other sounds. Once the Hum had captured Jody's attention, she couldn't focus on anything else or hold anything in mind. The Hum made Jody's attention difficulties worse than they had been.

It sounded as though the Hum was outside of her body and Jody was constantly searching for it. But then she realised that she could hear the Hum everywhere, and began to believe that it was inside her somehow. Jody hated this idea and was frightened.

Jody couldn't sleep with the sound of the Hum, or rest or read in a quiet place. She could not escape it, and she was distressed and exhausted. Jody felt trapped with the Hum, and did not understand it, especially as other people could not hear it. Jody stopped talking about it, but then felt more isolated and alone with the Hum.

Jody fought against the idea that the Hum was inside her. She tried not to think about it but this only made her more aware of it. This was unusual for Jody, who had been able to accept many of the first stroke changes.

What was the Hum?

The Hum may have been triggered by Jody's second bleed or the stress it caused. The sound may have been inside her brain, or caused by an unusual perception of a low frequency sound in the outside world. Whether the sound came from outside or not, it seems to have been caused by a change in Jody's brain that allowed her to hear the Hum.

Some people can develop an extra sensitivity to low frequency sounds that others cannot hear. This ability to hear these sounds as a low rumble or hum is not fully understood. The sound travels through the air for several miles and it is very difficult to pinpoint where it is coming from.

Most people never find the source of the sound. A sensitivity to low frequency noise coming from an industrial site some distance away might explain why Jody could hear it all the time, wherever she went.

Jody had noticed sounds and other unusual sensations inside her head since the first stroke. She often heard clicking and banging sounds and experienced fizzing sensations. The Hum may have been caused by an extra sensitivity to 'hearing' activity in Jody's brain.

Other people's experience

Being unable to escape from a constant unpleasant sound can cause physical and mental health problems. Unidentified sounds can be frightening, and can trigger a red alert state of stress and anxiety.

Finding the source of the sound can become an obsession, as Jody described. There is no one to be angry and frustrated with if the source of the sound cannot be traced. People can become low in mood because they don't understand the sound and can't control it.

People often feel very negative about sounds like the Hum. The distress it causes and the desire to escape it can dominate their lives, and even limit what people do and where they go.

Beliefs about the sound, where it is coming from and who could switch it off can also be very powerful. These negative interpretations, and the uncertainty and powerlessness involved, can be as distressing as the sound itself.

> ### Things that can help
>
> Jody was told that she did not have tinnitus, but that she might benefit from things that help with tinnitus.
>
> Understanding tinnitus and having support from people with experience of it can reduce the stress, even if the sound does not change. Tinnitus organisations have books, websites and training programs dedicated to helping people to cope.
>
> Silence can make the tinnitus sound seem louder. Background sound can help to mask it. Having the radio or TV on in the background, or music playing through headphones, can make the tinnitus less noticeable. Electric fans or a clock with a loud 'tick', recordings of nature sounds or white noise can also be used.
>
> The background sound should be pleasant or neutral and not too loud. There are special sound generators designed to help with tinnitus, mobile phone apps and special hearing aids that also play quiet sounds.
>
> Background sounds can be particularly helpful at night when things are quieter. Some people sleep with a window open so they can hear distant traffic, the wind and the rain. Background sound and relaxation routines at bedtime can help people go to sleep, and to sleep better.
>
> The distress caused by tinnitus or low frequency sound can improve when people change the way they respond to it. This can be a difficult step, but is often very helpful. Following a relaxation program can help because stress can make tinnitus worse.
>
> Relaxation can make the sound seem quieter and help people to focus on something else. Being busy and involved in things can also help – because attention is focused on something more positive than the sound.
>
> Professional support can be helpful if worry, stress, anxiety and depression are severe. It may help to become more aware of negative thoughts about the tinnitus, because these tend to increase anxiety and low mood. There are also programmes designed to retrain the brain's response to sound, so that the tinnitus is less noticeable.
>
> Mindfulness can help with tinnitus by drawing attention away from the tinnitus and making the person more aware of other sounds. Or, bringing a greater acceptance to the tinnitus, allowing it to be as it is, may bring the most benefit in the long run. Jody found it very difficult to bring acceptance to the Hum when she first had it, perhaps because she was going through a particularly difficult time.

Coming to Terms with a Stroke or Brain Injury

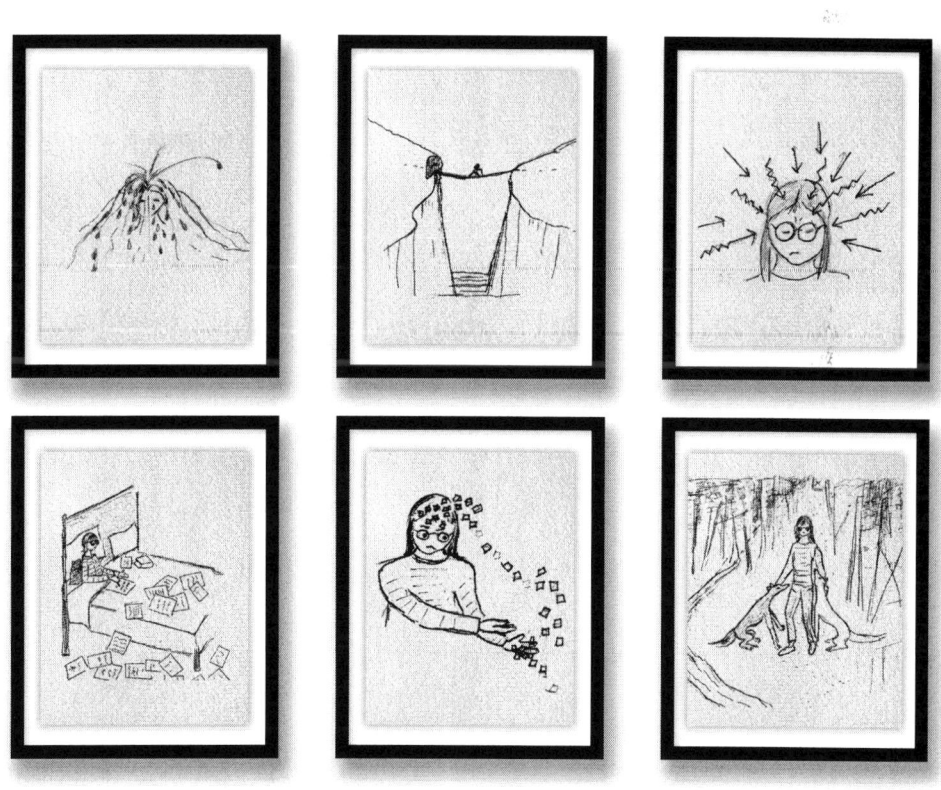

Chapter 34: Loss, Grief and Emotional Distress

A stroke or brain injury creates many losses. Some of these may be visible and obvious – the loss of mobility, the loss of work and income, the loss of a driving licence – clear evidence of the impact of the brain injury. These are also potent reminders of the person's loss of independence, which can be one of the most significant losses of a brain injury.

Other losses may be less obvious. Relationships, responsibilities and roles can all change in subtle ways. A brain injury often reduces the person's sense of self-control – the ability to control their body, their mind, their behaviour and emotions, and the direction of their life.

The person may be aware of the changes and experience the loss directly. Others may be less aware of how they have changed, but will know that something is missing and not right. This causes bewilderment and confusion as well as sadness.

Jody's experience of loss

Jody described many instances of loss. Many were about the loss of ability. Others were losses in Jody's relationships with people, and in her identity and sense of self.

Loss of ability

Jody's cognitive abilities had changed. 'How busy and inventive my brain was. I didn't know how important all that was until I lost it' (Chapter 5). Jody struggled to cope without the smooth, efficient running of her brain. Everything required more effort and time.

Jody was less independent generally, and travelling independently was particularly difficult. She had travelled alone since she was very young, and her independence had been important.

Jody lost confidence in her body and her mind. She could not trust her body to stay balanced or to keep going. Brain crashes and memory slips seemed to arrive suddenly.

Working life

Jody had many different responsibilities and roles in her working life. She returned to most of these after the first stroke, but had to let go of them again after the second one.

Giving up her job as Director of the mindfulness centre created a huge loss. The job had given her status and influence, work satisfaction and contact with people. Later, and sometimes with great sadness, Jody gradually let go of her other professional roles.

Relationship changes

Connection with people

Jody met with much love, support and kindness during her recovery – from her family, friends, colleagues and strangers. But as she recovered, she realised she could not connect in the same way with the people she knew well. Being with people she knew well reminded Jody of how much she had changed.

Other people don't always understand

Jody felt that other people did not understand her difficulties. With the kindest of intentions, friends reassured Jody that they too had 'senior moments' and memory lapses. It was hard for her to convey that her memory problems were different and more severe. It was particularly difficult for people to understand how things slipped from her mind without warning.

Understanding the misunderstanding

It was obvious to people that Jody had changed when she was confused or forgetful. It was less obvious that she felt different all of the time, that she was always struggling to cope and to get things right. Jody was aware that people didn't know this. She understood that they could not see her invisible difficulties, and the constant effort of coping with them.

Other people reassured Jody, and looked for improvements. They wanted her to be the same as she was before. Jody knew this was impossible – she had changed so much.

A difficult journey for everyone

Jody could see how difficult it was for other people – she was the same, and yet different. Who was Jody now? Everyone was asking the same question. Unexpected sudden changes in a person's identity and sense of self strike at the heart of relationships, which, despite everyone's best efforts, cannot be the same again.

A friend with the same viewpoint

Jody was often more comfortable with people who did not know her before her stroke. A new friendship was a fresh start. She enjoyed talking to strangers. They could not compare her with how she was before.

Jody had a friend with a similar brain injury and their shared understanding was comforting. They both knew about a different way of relating to the world, and the 'new normal'.

A smaller social life

Jody's difficulties limited her social activities. She couldn't go for long walks with family and friends, and many indoor places were too loud, busy and overwhelming for Jody to manage. She stayed at home a lot more.

Jody could not cope with social gatherings in the early months. She could not keep up with conversations. Playing board games made it easier to be with people, and on an equal footing with them. The rules of the game were helpful when she couldn't follow the rules of conversation or understand jokes. Games allowed Jody to get close to people again, to have fun with them.

Family and close friends

Jody described the changes in her relationship with family and friends as her 'greatest loss and sadness' (Chapter 17). It was 'terribly hard and often heart wrenching to be with people I loved' (Chapter 7).

Jody's family and friends had to get to know her again, as a different person. She knew she could not be the same mother because she was not the same person, and that her family felt the loss of her. Although Jody was content to be different at other times, she longed to be her old self when she was with her family.

There was a break in the continuity of Jody's relationship with the world. We expect people and relationships to feel stable and permanent, and it is deeply disturbing when they change.

The impact of the second stroke

Old and new difficulties

Jody had worked hard to regain lost ground after the first stroke, but some difficulties either returned or were worse after the second. She also had the Hum to deal with. Jody again lost some of her ability to practice mindfulness – it seemed 'less deep, less regular' (Chapter 17). This was a significant loss at this difficult time.

Confidence in relationships

The second stroke was less severe, medically at least, and the changes were less obvious than the first time. However, Jody felt less understood, to the point of feeling invisible, a ghost of her former self. The second bleed had a huge impact on Jody's mood and view of herself.

Before the second stroke, Jody was usually happy to ask for help without doubting herself or others. But after the second stroke, she was anxious about being seen as a burden, or as a nuisance who was making a fuss unnecessarily. Jody had lost her confidence. She began to pretend that things were all right and to move further away from people.

A greater awareness of loss

There was a much deeper sense of loss around the effects of the second stroke. Jody experienced another shift in her sense of self. She was not the same person, for the second time, and this time it was not okay. She was also more aware of her difficulties and how they affected her life.

Misunderstanding and negative thinking

No one, including Jody, expected the impact of her second bleed to be significant. It was not a serious stroke. Everyone imagined that she would bounce back, with her usual resilience. The reality was quite different, but discovering this and attempting to cope with the new changes was a much more private affair the second time around.

Jody felt self-conscious and anxious about her difficulties. She did not like them or understand them. She felt she should have been doing better, and was slightly ashamed. Jody felt less motivated to regain her skills and knowledge. Everything required a huge effort, and was exhausting. This made everything in life feel more difficult.

Jody knew that the consequences of the second bleed were more difficult for people to understand. She knew that she appeared to be coping and getting better – but she was struggling with a growing sense of failure. People could not understand, and Jody stopped trying to explain. This pushed her deeper into a dark and lonely place.

Adjusting to loss after a brain injury

How easily a person adjusts to a brain injury will depend on many different influences. Their personality and past experience will shape how they respond to their difficulties. Some longstanding patterns are more helpful than others. Jody's mindfulness practice, and the way she could bring acceptance to her difficulties after the first stroke, calmed her, preserved her energy and helped her to keep going.

Emotional well-being also depends on the person's situation and surroundings. If someone is unrealistic, and trying to recreate the demanding life they had before their brain injury, they will be distressed and stressed, and possibly depressed and anxious.

But if they are no longer trying to achieve the impossible, their home is adapted and their family understands and supports them, the same person, with the same brain injury, may have relatively few emotional difficulties. Unfortunately, this ideal is hard to achieve in real-life situations, which are often very complex and difficult to manage.

All aspects of an injured person's circumstances can affect their psychological health; working out what causes distress and changing key aspects of the situation can help enormously.

Although Jody's second stroke was less severe than the first, the changes it caused were more difficult to adjust to. Amongst the losses of the first stroke, Jody had gained a new perspective and some new gifts, such as 'new eyes' and a strong sense of connection with people. Adjusting to the loss of these after the second stroke was perhaps the greatest challenge of all.

Psychological responses to a brain injury

People often have a strong emotional reaction to their brain injury and the losses involved. Unfortunately, these normal emotional responses can easily escalate after a brain injury. They often develop into more severe conditions that almost have a life of their own, and cannot be snapped out of. Many people with a brain injury develop clinical depression and anxiety states.

Jody was mildly depressed and generally more anxious for a while after the second stroke. The tranquillity and acceptance she experienced after her first stroke had largely disappeared. Jody had unpredictable shifts in her mood and perspective. She was worried and fearful about the future, and there was a sense of things closing in around her. Her mood was low and she seemed resigned rather than accepting.

Depression: what is it?

Depression is the most common emotional complication of a stroke or brain injury. The main symptoms of depression include low mood, loss of pleasure and interest, low self-esteem and memory and concentration problems. People also develop negative thinking patterns and can be wrapped up in feelings of guilt, worthlessness and inadequacy.

Physical symptoms include fatigue, poor sleep, appetite and weight changes, restlessness or lethargy. These symptoms tend to be severe, stable and long-lasting.

What can cause depression after brain injury?

Depression is often a reaction to the person's awareness of their disabilities, and to the losses their injury has caused. For some people, depression is also directly related to their physical brain injury changes.

Depression is very common after a stroke. However, people with a stroke on the left side of their brain are more likely to become depressed in the early months of recovery than people who have a stroke on the right side of their brain. This is because they tend to be more immediately aware of the effects of the stroke.

How does depression develop?

The symptoms and difficulties caused by any brain injury can be very frightening at first. The person may have severe physical difficulties, as well as bewildering cognitive and emotional changes.

The person is likely to feel very concerned about the future, about whether they will get better, and by how much. If and when it becomes clear that progress will be slow or that some things may never improve, low mood and depression may well develop.

People can feel very angry and very frustrated by their limitations. The lack of control over their own life can make people feel helpless and hopeless, and wear away at their self-confidence and self-esteem.

Motivation and energy

Motivation, energy and stamina can be reduced by a brain injury and by depression. If a person has both a brain injury and depression, there may be a double decline.

Depression is likely to interfere with rehabilitation efforts. Physiotherapy, attending groups and trying to be more active can take more energy and drive than the person has. Other people may not be able to raise the person's energy or enthusiasm levels, which can be discouraging and cause further difficulty.

Is it depression or 'just' the brain injury?

Many of the symptoms of depression overlap with brain injury difficulties. Fatigue, poor sleep, lack of energy and interest, being slowed down, memory and concentration problems and feeling irritable are problems shared by brain injury and depression. It can be difficult to tell the difference between them, and to know whether someone with a brain injury is also depressed.

Clinical depression is not the same as feeling low or unhappy because of the stroke or brain injury. These normal responses become much more intense when depression develops, and the symptoms last for longer when someone is depressed.

Depression holds back recovery and increases difficulty

Having depression as well as a brain injury makes existing problems worse. Recovery is slower and people benefit less from rehabilitation when they have depression as well as a brain injury. This does not depend on how severe the injury is – depression increases difficulty for everyone who has a brain injury.

Depression impacts on family relationships at a time when family care and support is most needed. Depression, which often goes together with anxiety, can be a barrier to recovery.

Recovery from depression

Depression often improves over time as the person learns to live with their difficulties. However, emotional distress and depression can also stand still or get worse over time, and it is important that others are aware of the injured person's moods and emotions. Depression and brain injury carry the risk of desperate distress. Suicidal thoughts and suicide attempts by people with a brain injury, especially a TBI, are not uncommon.

Ways of helping

Depression can be treated with antidepressant medication, or with talking therapies, or both. It can be a relief to discuss fears, despair, loss and grief openly and without fear of judgement in a therapy session, and to try to make sense of what has happened.

Therapy can help us to learn new ways of thinking about the situation, and new ways of coping with difficulty. It can help us decide what we want to work towards, and how to break that down into smaller, achievable goals. Making progress, being more involved in things and creating more opportunity for enjoyment can help to reduce depression symptoms.

Mindfulness based cognitive therapy for depression is known to be helpful. Learning to practice mindfulness has been shown to help people who are depressed and anxious after a brain injury.

Getting out and about, doing more and having opportunities for enjoyment can also help a great deal. Gaining satisfaction and pleasure from things, boosting self-esteem and confidence, can help to overcome low mood and negative thinking. Physical activity in itself has a powerful antidepressant effect. It is important to be as active as possible, within the injury's limitations.

Anxiety

What causes anxiety after a brain injury?
Anxiety is a natural reaction to the frightening effects of a brain injury, and is almost as common as depression. An injury can create traumatic memories and the fear that it might happen again. People are often anxious about having another stroke; a brain injury in a car accident can lead to a fear of road travel.

There is often anxiety about the future and what lies ahead. The experience of being less able than before erodes self-confidence and creates a fear of not being able to cope.

Anxiety can rule our lives (if we let it)
Fear of not coping can make us want to escape or hide away – and it can trigger a vicious cycle of anxiety and avoidance. We may feel better when we escape or hide, but we lose the chance to discover that we might have coped after all. Hiding away also makes us more anxious in the long run, and then we want to hide away even more.

The long term effects of hiding away – avoiding difficulties and escaping from fear – are usually negative. Avoiding anxiety also means avoiding opportunities in life, for getting out and about, and perhaps enjoying things. With reassurance and support, aiming to do more rather than hide away is likely to help in the long run.

What is anxiety?
The most obvious signs of anxiety are felt in the body, and are often mistaken for a physical illness. In its most extreme form, anxiety can cause a panic attack, which can feel like a heart attack or a sudden breathing problem. Inevitably, feeling as though we are about to die makes anxiety even worse.

The physical signs of anxiety include sweating, a racing heart, breathing difficulties and feeling lightheaded, dizzy and faint. There can be tension in the muscles, leading to cramps, aches and pains. Anxiety also plays havoc with the digestive system: people often feel sick, cannot eat properly or develop bowel symptoms, including cramping and diarrhoea.

Anxiety causes sleep problems – either trouble with going to sleep or staying asleep. Worrying at night is very common, and poor sleep leads to further exhaustion and fatigue.

Concentrating, thinking clearly and making decisions are more difficult when people are anxious. The person may also be restless, perhaps pacing up and down, and they may be more irritable.

Extreme worry, especially about the future, is a hallmark of anxiety. Severe anxiety often involves irrational fears and phobias, as well as realistic concerns about a difficult situation. We can worry about our anxiety and how to get rid of it, and become anxious about being anxious.

Panic attacks are not life-threatening but they are very unpleasant, and something that people want to avoid. Again, this can lead to avoidance of situations, people and doing difficult things. Fear about being among people is one of the most common forms of anxiety after a brain injury.

People with a brain injury who are very anxious about their difficulties sometimes have emotional outbursts that might be described as 'meltdowns'. They can involve intense distress and long episodes of crying. These catastrophic reactions often stem from anxiety about the effects of the stroke or brain injury, when the difficulties have not yet been acknowledged or accepted by the injured person.

Brain injury and anxiety also overlap

Some of the symptoms of anxiety are so similar to brain injury problems that they can be hard to tell apart. A brain injury and anxiety can both cause fatigue, restlessness and irritability, dizziness, trembling, poor concentration and a sense of unreality and detachment from the world.

A loss of confidence and realistic worries and concerns about the future after a brain injury are not the same as an anxiety condition.

From cotton wool to a tightrope

Care and support after the injury usually begins with medical and nursing care. Relatives and professionals often provide care at home later. The person is likely to be dependent on others for some time.

As recovery continues, taking steps towards greater independence can trigger high levels of anxiety for everyone involved. The injured person may not want to try new things – they may be afraid of falling, of failing, of embarrassing themselves and being seen as disabled.

It is natural for caregivers to protect the injured person from risk of further injury, failure and more distress. Wanting to wrap them in cotton wool is normal and natural. However, cotton wool doesn't allow much room for improvement; the understandable anxiety and avoidance needs to be balanced against regaining as much independence as possible.

Recovery and rehabilitation involves gradually doing more and becoming more independent. This can feel like stepping out on a tightrope, or onto Jody's rope bridge – wobbly, high and very scary. Taking small steps forwards increases the chances of growing success and regaining self-confidence gradually.

Trying to do too much can lead to failure and more anxiety, as well as disappointment and frustration. It's much harder to recover and to regain confidence after a setback than it is to aim for gradual progress and success in small steps. Unfortunately, people can be unrealistic about what they can do, and anxious at the same time, and so it can be hard to achieve a balance.

> ### Things that can help with anxiety
>
> Anxiety does not usually get better on its own, in the way that depression can, and professional support can be helpful. Anxiety can be improved in a number of different ways.
>
> Understanding what anxiety is, and what causes it, can bring huge relief. Information about anxiety can be very reassuring.
>
> It can be helpful to talk about what the fears and anxieties mean to the injured person and where they come from. Making sense of anxiety can make it feel less overwhelming, and reduce anxiety about getting anxious.
>
> Learning to relax can be very helpful. Taking time out with a relaxation or meditation recording. Learning to relax without using medication, alcohol or other drugs can make people feel more in control and able to cope with fearful situations.
>
> Gradually learning to cope with things that cause fear and anxiety is another helpful tactic. Try things out step by step.
>
> When anxiety is about what may happen in the future, focusing on the here and now can help. The problem usually isn't here right now.
>
> You could decide to cross that bridge when you come to it – you don't know that it will happen – or make plans for dealing with the situation if and when it happens. This can also reduce anxiety.
>
> Practicing and rebuilding old skills, being as active as possible and spending time with people who understand the situation can improve confidence and reduce anxiety about the future. It may be helpful to set small and realistic goals so that improvement is more visible. With some support, people with a stroke or brain injury can become more independent, despite feeling anxious.

Summary

Many people with a brain injury have depression or anxiety, regardless of how severe or mild the injury is.

Depression and anxiety can make existing memory and concentration problems worse. At the same time, depression and anxiety symptoms can be lost among the similar difficulties caused by the brain injury. It's important for other people to be aware of this.

If someone is struggling after a brain injury, depression and/or anxiety might be the cause.

Grief – connecting loss and sadness

Not everyone with a brain injury becomes depressed or anxious. However, everyone is likely to have some difficult emotional responses to the loss and change involved. These happen at different times and in different ways.

Emotional changes after a stroke or brain injury can be thought of as a grieving process. Grief is a natural response to any significant loss. It involves a complex procession of emotions and responses, beginning with shock, distress, sadness and anger, moving through these stages until the person can come to terms with their loss.

The aftermath of a brain injury can be like a bereavement. This idea can help us to understand what the injured person is going through, and what their family may be feeling about their loss.

Most people with a brain injury grieve in some way and at some time for the things they have lost. Grief and sadness can be particularly intense if the injured person feels that they have changed in themselves.

Grief after a brain injury is more complicated than a bereavement in many ways. No one has passed away. There is no funeral or public recognition of the loss, only hope for further recovery. The grieving process is also complicated by the cognitive and emotional changes caused by the brain injury, which can reduce the injured person's ability to understand their losses.

Grieving involves a lot of distress and intense emotion. Expressing these emotions and linking them to the losses may help the person to understand what has happened to them, and perhaps begin to come to terms with it. Understanding where these feelings come from is very helpful.

Understanding more about their brain injury and making sense of what has happened can also help the person to express their grief. Once grieving begins, it can help to move the injured person and their family towards an acceptance of their losses, even if this takes a long time and they need some help to get there.

Delayed grief

Loss and grief usually go together. When a loved one dies, the grieving process begins straight away. It may be delayed in some special circumstances – when a person is missing and is thought to have died, for instance. Grief cannot begin until a body is found or the uncertainty is resolved by the passage of time.

There is a parallel between a missing person and a person with a brain injury. Much of the early recovery can be spent waiting to see whether the injured person will come back as they were before. Relatives, in particular, may live with this uncertainty for many months, and grief may be on hold until the question is resolved.

Grief may be delayed for other reasons too. It takes time for the person to become aware of their difficulties, to accept them and to include their brain injury as part of their new identity. Grief cannot begin in earnest until these processes are underway. These stages are all part of adjusting to the injury.

Coming to terms with the injury

Adjusting to a stroke or brain injury involves working through emotions about it and making changes along the way – developing self-awareness of the difficulties, making sense of the losses, becoming more accepting of them and grieving.

Unfortunately, these adjustments can be extremely challenging and there are many potential obstacles along the way. The obstacles may be linked directly to the brain injury – for example, inflexible thinking or having little awareness of the difficulties caused by the stroke. Or they may stem from the psychological trauma of being changed by the injury, such as denial, anger and bitterness.

Being unable to take these steps towards adjustment can lead to a situation that feels very stuck. The person may be caught up in a battle with their injury and their emotions. This can also result in depression or anxiety, which is another layer of difficulty to cope with.

Summary

A stroke or brain injury causes losses of many kinds – from the loss of independent mobility to the loss of humour and spontaneity. Grief is a natural response to any significant loss, including the loss of a person as they were, through the injury.

People with a brain injury and their families may go through a long process of grieving, moving from early stages of shock, denial, sadness and anger to greater acceptance and long-term adjustment. However, as we shall see, this process can only lead to adjustment if the injured person is aware of their difficulties, and can eventually include their stroke or brain injury as part of their new identity.

Things that can help

Talking about the losses and expressing sadness and grief can be very helpful if the person is ready to do this.

The person with the injury may need help with thinking about what they have lost and how they feel about it. Talking about this kind of thing may be more difficult for them than it was before the injury.

It is important that the person discusses their difficulties and their emotions only when they are ready to. Pushing too hard can cause overwhelming emotions and reactions that are best avoided.

Chapter 35: The Problem of Reduced Self-Awareness

It can take a long time after a stroke or brain injury for the person to discover how it has affected them. They may be in a coma or not fully conscious for a long time, and then unwell, confused and disoriented.

As they begin to get better, the person will start to discover what they can and cannot do. A brain injury can affect many different abilities, and it takes time to find out what has changed. Problems with more difficult tasks will only be discovered later.

Some people cannot see how they have been affected – because they have reduced self-awareness of their difficulties. This confusing complication is very common straight after the injury, particularly after a stroke on the right side of the brain. It can clear up within days or weeks. However, some people have a severe and long-term difficulty with self-awareness. Caring for someone with this problem can be very challenging.

The 'blind spot' may be part of the injury itself. The parts of the brain that allow us to know ourselves and our strengths and weaknesses are often affected by an injury. The main issue is that people are unrealistic, and unable to appreciate their own need for support. Reduced self-awareness may turn into a permanent disability, and can be a major stumbling block for rehabilitation.

The person may believe that they are doing well, and may refuse help and support. They may try to resume activities that they cannot manage, such as driving or working, oblivious to safety issues and the likelihood of failure. They may take unreasonable risks. People with reduced self-awareness cannot anticipate problems or judge how things will turn out, and these difficulties are often played out over and over again.

People may focus on their physical disabilities, and accept help with them, while being unaware of cognitive, emotional and behavioural changes. This can be a huge barrier to engaging with therapy and rehabilitation, and to living as well as possible.

The causes of reduced self-awareness are not properly understood. They can stem from physical changes in the brain, especially injury to the front of the brain. Self-awareness is a complex executive ability in itself. People with reduced self-awareness often have other executive problems – they may be inflexible, or show little sympathy, or have little understanding of other people's point of view.

The most severe brain injuries cause the most difficulty. Most people have some degree of self-awareness, and this causes fewer problems.

Reduced self-awareness may also be an emotional reaction to the injury. The person may be in denial about their injury, unconsciously trying to protect themselves from the distress they would feel if they acknowledged it.

People with reduced self-awareness are more disadvantaged than others, partly because they do not want to take part in rehabilitation. They are less likely to return to work successfully or to have positive relationships with family and friends. Reduced self-awareness causes stress in family life. Families want to protect their injured relative from their unrealistic decisions and risky behaviour.

Reduced self-awareness is a complex and perplexing aspect of brain injury. It can be severe and very limiting, or so subtle that it is never fully recognised. It can be very difficult for other people to understand. Relatives and professionals may all struggle to pinpoint the problem and how it is causing further difficulties.

Jody's self-awareness – after the first stroke

Some of Jody's problems were immediately obvious to her. She knew 'without thought' that something fundamental had changed and that she was not the same person. Jody had 'no idea' how much the stroke had affected her at first, and would have been terrified if she had known: 'I don't think I realised I had a brain injury then' (Chapter 4).

But she knew from the start that she did not know herself, and that she needed to find out how she was and who she was now. Jody commented that the many consequences of her brain injury were not the ones she might have imagined (Chapter 1).

Jody's awareness of her difficulties developed slowly. As she tried to do more, she encountered new problems. However, she continued to experience her difficulties as if for the first time. The stroke had affected Jody more than she thought – and she had this realisation many times over.

Jody didn't realise there were more changes to discover. It took several years for Jody to fully understand the effects of her stroke, and to be able to explain it to other people.

Jody's growing self-awareness of her difficulties

Jody was immediately aware of physical changes – problems with walking and balance, and with visual perception. Jody gradually realised that her memory was poor and she couldn't remember the names of things she knew well.

Changes in planning and organisation took much longer to recognise, along with subtle changes in Jody's behaviour. Planning and self-awareness are controlled by overlapping brain networks. If our executive functions are injured, our self-awareness tends to suffer too.

Self-awareness after brain injury usually develops in this way. It begins with physical problems. Awareness of more subtle and complex problems tends to develop later.

Awareness through the present moment

In the first few weeks of her recovery, Jody's stroke symptoms and the outside world were bewildering and alien. She was comforted by her inner world of moment by moment experience. Jody imagined at the time that this was how she would make sense of her stroke – that she would understand it through her inner experience. 'And who am I – this question of who am I... I am just my experience – and that seems enough' (Chapter 8).

Despite its benefits, Jody's present moment experience did not allow her to become aware of her difficulties. She could not remember her moment by moment experience clearly. It did not help her to build a picture of how she was in the world now – or create an explanation that she could talk about.

Looking back, Jody describes this stage very clearly. 'I understood myself from how I was Being, was experiencing my life – mapped it all out in pictures – found it in poems' (Chapter 7). This helped me to understand why Jody's awareness of her difficulties was not mapped out in words, as I might have expected, given her gift for writing and reflection.

People make sense of what has happened to them in different ways, and may not be able to describe it in words.

Jody's 'new eyes'

Jody always described the experience of her difficulties very clearly. But she wrote little about their impact on her life, or how she made sense of them.

Jody did not bring her experience together to form ideas and statements about her own difficulties. Her understanding of her experience was developing in a different way. Jody's 'new eyes' saw the world more clearly than before, but they were not connected to her thinking mind. Jody's new eyes and quiet mind could not turn her experience into words and descriptions at the time.

A turning point

Jody became aware that while she had been caught up in her dream-like world of Being, she was 'struggling with Doing… activities – with accessing my thinking and organising mind' (Chapter 7). She knew then that her recovery would depend on keeping 'the thinking part of me strong, not to succumb to the lure of just letting go and sensing'.

This moment of choice reflected a turning point in the development of Jody's self-awareness and her recovery. She began to use strategies to manage other problems – and was aware of how they were helping her.

Learning about difficulties in the real world

Jody's first train journeys and her visit to Brighton were another leap forward, and they revealed how much Jody had changed. 'The seeds of difficulties I was to encounter in returning to my world, life, family and work were there in that early Brighton visit' (Chapter 5). Jody learned about memory problems she had not recognised, and found that she had lost talents that were important to her. Some of these discoveries were hard to take.

Jody started doing more, and doing more demanding things. Unfortunately, this revealed more difficulty, and Jody sometimes felt that she was 'getting worse'. When Jody went back to work, new difficulties with memory, perception, fatigue and relationships all surfaced.

Jody became less attuned to her physical sensations and became more aware of her mind. This was an essential part of Jody's growing awareness of her difficulties.

Coping, concern and curiosity

Jody was often more curious than concerned about the impact of her stroke. She noted that other people were 'far more concerned by apparent changes in me than I ever have been' (Chapter 8).

Jody did have moments of concern, of course. After coming across new problems in Brighton, she was very concerned about whether she could cope at the family weddings or back at work. And for the first time she was uneasy about what people thought of her.

Jody often felt anxious and concerned when she was confused or overwhelmed. She learned to cope with this by staying present. Jody told herself not to engage with panicky thoughts. She realised that she could disconnect the 'trying to think' part of her brain and that this would calm her.

Nevertheless, Jody felt less concern about her stroke and was less worried about the future than people often expected. This was most obvious when things were calm and stable. Jody was not living in her mind with thoughts and worries. There was no background of continuous concern. Jody was much more absorbed in what she was doing at the time.

Jody's contentment and lack of concern came partly from the attitude of acceptance that she cultivated. But it may also have stemmed from her reduced self-awareness of her difficulties.

Motivation to improve

Many people with incomplete self-awareness or lack of concern have problems with the idea of rehabilitation. Jody had the opposite attitude. She was consistently motivated to make progress and worked hard to improve her situation.

Understanding the impact of difficulties on life

There is a difference between knowing what the difficulties are and understanding how they will affect daily life. Many people with a brain injury can name their difficulties without necessarily seeing how they will change things.

Jody was willing and able to recognise many of her difficulties and could see how they had changed things. She knew how difficult it had been for her to organise things at home. She could see the effects of her difficulties when she looked back, but she could not anticipate their effects in the future. Jody was not fully aware of the implications of her difficulties.

It was hard for Jody to learn from mistakes and difficulties in the past. Imagine that we have a special log book in our memory where we record what we have done, what has worked and what has gone wrong. This record allows us to predict what will work again in the future and to know what we should avoid. It was as though Jody's brain did not write in this log book – or did not look back at it to see what had gone wrong in the past. As a result, she had difficulty learning about her strengths and her weaknesses.

Anticipating problems

Jody was often surprised by her difficulties and rarely predicted problems in advance. Jody did not expect the walls, trees and lampposts to move, and for things to look different. When she visited Brighton for the second time, Jody was surprised to have the same difficulties as before. She half expected that things would be back to normal.

Jody was shocked when her brain crashed during the mindfulness conference. She began to realise that she should avoid certain places and situations, that she needed to pace herself and not do too much. She tried to learn how far she could push herself – how far she could drive safely before she needed to rest.

These were not easy lessons. Jody had many crashes before she remembered what to avoid, and before she could recognise the first physical and mental signs of a crash or her memory slipping. 'I find that now all these years on, I am better at this game with my mind – I know this, ah, I think, I can feel the slipping sensation, something is going.' Jody also learned to remind herself that this had happened before (Chapter 21).

Awareness through stories and images

Jody's self-awareness of her difficulties is expressed most clearly through the images she drew and wrote about in her journals: the tsunami of blood raging through her brain, and the orange bowl that could hold only one or two ideas. It was easier for Jody to express her understanding of herself through these images, rather than through factual descriptions.

An image of something physical made her difficulties more real. They helped Jody to be more aware of them and to make sense of them. She also described them to her colleagues, to help them to understand the problems too.

Several years after her stroke, Jody was not always aware that her mind would empty if she added another orange to the bowl. This shows how difficult it was for her to learn about her difficulties. Jody used the orange bowl idea to remind herself that this would happen, but it took years to learn to do this.

Jody's story of her journey and the map she has drawn vividly expresses her self-awareness and her understanding of the stroke. It highlights Jody's realisation that she could not go back, and her awareness of the unknown challenges that lay ahead.

Jody could not explain her difficulties in words. But her description of her slow, step by step progress across the rope bridge, high above the sea, communicates her clear perception of the profound changes in her life and the emotions that came with them.

Summary: after the first stroke
Jody had difficulty understanding and holding onto a clear picture of her brain injury changes. She could identify the individual changes, but could not combine them, to see the 'bigger picture'.

Her memory problems may have contributed to this, but her reduced self-awareness was more complicated than not remembering what her difficulties were. She could not see what the impact of her difficulties would be. Her problems surprised her and she could not predict them. She often experienced difficulties as if for the first time.

Jody's self-awareness improved gradually. The story of her journey, and thinking about her difficulties as physical objects and events, helped her to make sense of her experience. Jody also understood her injury in terms of the strategies that worked for her.

A person with a brain injury may not be able to describe exactly what the problem is, but they may know what helps them and what they need other people to do.

The second lightning strike – further changes in self-awareness
Jody's description of her difficulties after the second stroke had a different quality. She had a wider and more direct awareness of her difficulties. They were more joined up, and less like separate problems.

This new awareness seemed to develop quite abruptly, unlike the slow, gradual development of awareness the first time. Jody was more aware of the impact of the difficulties, and her awareness was perhaps more realistic.

Jody's awareness of loss and low mood
Jody's new awareness was also more negative. She wrote a lot about loss and sadness, and her mood was lower than before. There was dislike rather than acceptance in her writing.

She began to realise that her brain injury changes might be permanent, and was frightened by that idea. She could see how much ability and knowledge had been 'washed away' by both of her haemorrhages. She knew that these could not be regained.

The powerful image of Jody and her abilities fragmenting and becoming a jigsaw puzzle reveals an acute awareness of her difficulties and the lack of control she had over them. 'Some days I can move some pieces, others I just pack them away in a box' (Chapter 16).

Self-awareness and depression

We know that self-awareness and mood affect each other. Becoming more aware of difficulties can lead to depression – people who don't know about their difficulties may be protected from becoming depressed about them.

After her first stroke, Jody was not fully aware of her difficulties, and she was not depressed. After the second stroke, she was more aware of her difficulties, and her mood was lower.

It seems unlikely that the second stroke increased Jody's self-awareness – strokes usually make things worse. It is more likely that her low mood was a natural response to the setback of the second stroke, and that the shift in her mood made her more aware of her difficulties. The connection between self-awareness and depression after brain injury is complex – changes in awareness can affect mood; changes in mood can affect awareness.

Low mood is something to look out for in a person who is becoming more aware of their brain injury difficulties.

Understanding her brain injury

For many months and even years, Jody felt that she was finding out about her brain injury for the first time. She learned about her stroke with H, her clinical neuropsychologist. However, when Jody and I talked about it later, she responded to the same information as if it was new. Her surprise and interest demonstrated how little she had been able to absorb about her difficulties.

Jody may not have remembered what H had said, or have known how to make sense of it.

When Jody talked about her stroke as a whole, she described it in very general terms, often referring to the idea that her experiences were normal in the sphere of brain injury.

Jody wrote several more times that she was discovering 'the territory of' brain injury. Close to the end of her story, Jody once again felt that she was beginning to understand her brain injury – as if she were a toddler 'seeing things for the first time' (Chapter 22). This also illustrates how difficult it can be for people with a stroke to become aware of their difficulties.

Jody's growing awareness of her difficulties

Towards the end of her story, Jody was acutely aware of her cognitive difficulties. She described the impact of her memory and organisation problems: 'the twin experience of forgetting and not being able to organise has such a great influence on how I manage life and work post haemorrhages.' The way that forgetting everything 'contributes to the chaos that can accompany me through life now' (Chapter 21).

Jody recognised problems with the control of her memory and the way that memory is organised and searched. 'My brain will not easily organise material... my memory has to go somewhere, be stored – it is almost as if I am in an office with piles of paper but nowhere to put them' (Chapter 21).

She described 'constantly putting paper into a nice, neat pile only for it to fall into a heap on the floor' (Chapter 21). Jody again used physical images to describe her experience. However, these statements reveal a new, more abstract awareness of the complex executive abilities described earlier. These include the structuring and organising of information, and an awareness of her awareness.

Changes in Jody's self-awareness: summary

Jody was aware of difficulties as they happened, and she described her experience of them in detail. But she could not see the bigger picture of her stroke or anticipate problems in daily life. This may explain why Jody was less concerned about her difficulties than other people were.

After the first stroke, Jody made sense of her difficulties most clearly through images, metaphors and poetry. She had more self-awareness after the second stroke. She could describe and make sense of her difficulties more easily.

Jody's difficulty with awareness was relatively subtle, and was not a barrier to her self-directed rehabilitation and recovery. The following section looks at more severe self-awareness problems, and how they are approached in a rehabilitation setting.

Developing self-awareness in rehabilitation

Supporting people with reduced self-awareness and helping them to improve their self-awareness is often a challenge. Providing information about their brain injury and giving genuine feedback about the person's difficulties can make a difference. For example, the results of rehabilitation assessments are often shared with the injured person and their family.

At the same time, people with reduced self-awareness may be fragile and may want to avoid talking about their difficulties. In this case, a gentle and sometimes sideways approach can be more helpful.

The desire to improve self-awareness is often at the heart of brain injury rehabilitation programmes because reduced self-awareness has such a negative impact on people's lives. Most of this involves information or education about brain injury or feedback about the person's strengths and weaknesses.

Brain injury education is usually taught in groups. Information is often presented in stories about other people – fictional characters with a stroke or brain injury. People in the group often identify with the characters, and may begin to recognise some of their own problems.

One of the best ways forward is to ask the group what they would do to help the character in question. This can loosen up resistance to taking advice or making changes. The group will often begin to discuss their own strengths and weaknesses in relation to their new understanding of brain injury.

Meeting with people who have similar difficulties can be a key to developing self-awareness. This may be a social group, or a brain injury education group, or perhaps group work on a DIY or gardening project. Groups like this are sometimes run in the voluntary sector – by Headway and the Stroke Association, for example.[2]

Focusing on an activity rather than problems can also be helpful. It is important that information and feedback are given in a supportive situation, by people who are already trusted. Members of the group can support each other and talk about themselves together, and this can increase self-awareness more naturally.

Trying to challenge the person's beliefs about their brain injury is not usually helpful. Giving information or feedback and allowing people to move towards their own conclusions is usually more effective. If rehabilitation is available, taking part in activities and projects that are about building skills and making progress can be more positive than 'therapy' for problems the person doesn't recognise.

Talking therapy for people with reduced self-awareness can also be helpful. It is important to put the injured person's experience and viewpoint at the centre of the conversation, and to work together on the problems that they can recognise and face.

---

2 see Further Reading on p308 for links to these organisations.

It is important to move gently, to avoid pushing the person towards increased self-awareness before they are ready. Once the process has started, it can be useful to talk about the awareness problem itself, as long as this is done carefully and sensitively, and the person seems to be coping.

As we have seen in Jody's story, increased self-awareness can be linked to low mood and anxiety. This means that feedback should be gentle and consistent rather than challenging or confrontational. People with reduced self-awareness are often very fragile psychologically, and could have unhelpful overwhelming emotional reactions if they are forced to face difficulties too soon.

Summary

The problem of reduced self-awareness can range from mild and subtle to severe and disabling. Awareness usually improves over time, although some blind spots may never recover.

If you are involved with caring for someone with a brain injury, you may know about their difficulties before they do. Tread carefully when talking about them. They may be able to cope with some information or feedback, but could get angry or feel overwhelmed by too much at once.

People who are beginning to recognise their difficulties can feel vulnerable and anxious. They may feel angry, or hopeless and low. They may have extreme emotional outbursts.

People with reduced self-awareness may try to do more than they can cope with, and then be very frustrated and tired. Helping them to manage this can be very difficult.

Things that can help include:

Talking to the person about their brain injury. Asking them to say how it has affected them, and perhaps adding some further information. Building up a picture of the injury over time.

Discussing their strengths and their weaknesses – perhaps make a list. Thinking about how they would help someone else who had those problems, and prompt them if necessary. Thinking about how strengths might be used to improve weaknesses.

Playing games and doing activities that help concentration and memory. Making mistakes, being given feedback and seeing improvement can all help awareness to develop.

Giving gentle feedback at the time if something goes wrong – 'It happened because you couldn't remember the time of the appointment. You often forget things like that.'

Meeting other people with a brain injury can be helpful in many ways. Talking with others who have similar difficulties may allow the person to see those problems in themselves.

It is important to be sympathetic rather than blaming. You are giving feedback about something the person has no control over and cannot help.

continued >

If the person is rude or inappropriate without realising that they do this, give them feedback at the time, and talk about how you felt or how other people reacted.

If the person is unrealistic about something, but insists on being allowed to do it, it may be acceptable to let them try. It must be safe, and perhaps tried as a last resort. If they try and fail, they will need some help to get over it. It may help them to gain some awareness of the problem.

Reduced self-awareness can be a major obstacle in recovery from a stroke or brain injury. It needs to be treated with care, and not forced. The person is not closing their eyes or mind deliberately. It may be a direct result of the injury, or they may need more time to face their difficulties.

Chapter 36: Identity and Sense of Self

Shortly after her stroke, Jody looked in the mirror and realised that she was 'not the same'. She thought: 'this is like me… but not'. This sense of being changed has not disappeared. 'And I didn't know it then that this changed sense of self was going to be one of the major features of my life and recovering now… Somehow it changed everything' (Chapter 1).

Jody also went through the long process of discovering how the stroke had affected her, and of realising that she could not do things as she had done them before. Jody began to make changes to her identity, to eventually own the story of a new and different version of herself.

How does a brain injury affect a person's sense of self?

A person's identity is perhaps the biggest casualty of a brain injury. Our personal identity and sense of self are bound up with the continuous 'story of me'. It is our understanding of what we are like, what we are good at and how we came to be this way. It is based on our roles in life; it includes beliefs about how other people see us, and our future self. Our personal identity is tied closely to our self-confidence and self-esteem.

We are all strongly attached to our sense of self and to our personal identity – our strengths and our quirks, the things people like about us, and even the things they don't. We know these unique characteristics inside out. When they change, literally at a stroke, and the person does not know themselves any more, the impact is potentially devastating.

Many people with a brain injury are less able than they were before. Their behaviour, emotions and personality may also have altered. For most people, awareness of these changes is painful and distressing. Understandably, they want to be the way they were before. Rarely do people see brain injury changes in a positive light, especially at first.

What is more, having an altered sense of self goes against our fundamental need to be consistent and stable. We feel good about ourselves when we behave as others expect us to, and in a way that matches our sense of who we are. Significant 'then and now' changes in a person are a frightening threat to the continuity of their self, to who they are.

When a person's sense of self has been lost or changed, part of their recovery and adjustment lies in building a new and updated identity. This new sense of self needs to be linked to the old self, it cannot be completely different. Part of the new sense of self will be about what has changed, other parts will reflect what has stayed the same.

Comparing 'then and now'

When someone thinks about their brain injury, they will almost certainly compare themselves with how they were before. It is virtually impossible for people to avoid negative self-judgements, especially at first. We so often think less of ourselves when we are injured or compromised in some way, particularly when mental ability or emotional control are affected.

We may call ourselves 'stupid', 'ridiculous' or even 'crazy' when we make mistakes or get upset, and it is the same, but worse, after a brain injury. The person's message to their self may be 'you're not as good as you were' and 'not as good as you should be'. Self-esteem and self-confidence can plummet.

These comparisons can increase negative thoughts and feelings about being 'not as good'. This can be the beginning of a depressed way of thinking.

A lost sense of self

Many people lose touch with their sense of self after a brain injury. They literally don't know who they are anymore, and like Jody, they have to find out. They may be in a state of limbo between the old self and the new.

Their old identity no longer makes sense – the person has changed and the old 'me' doesn't apply any more. But the person may not yet know who the new 'me' is, and may be confused about their identity.

The situation is often held back by the emotional anguish and resistance involved in letting go of the old sense of self. We have a natural reluctance to replace the cherished old 'me' with an identity that may be less valued. Our minds were not designed to make a fundamental change in who we are.

A person might think: 'It's not like me to forget, or to be bad tempered – but if I am always forgetting and losing my temper, perhaps I am not me anymore? Or perhaps there is a new me who is forgetful and bad tempered?' This is all the more difficult when having a good memory or being even tempered are qualities that we value in ourselves.

Our inner self does not want 'me' to change in a negative way. Changing the picture of ourselves to include undesirable qualities is a threat to this sense of self. It creates a lot of anxiety. We may want to avoid and escape from this – perhaps through alcohol or drugs, or by hiding from the world.

A disconnected sense of self

It is not uncommon for a person to feel like a stranger to themselves after a brain injury. I worked with a young woman, Cathy, who felt completely disconnected from her old self and her life before her accident. She did not make 'then and now' comparisons because she could not remember herself as she was before her injury. Despite this disconnection, Cathy often had severe emotional reactions to anything related to her past skills and abilities.

Cathy often pushed herself beyond her limits, leading to exhaustion and several days in bed. She seemed unaware of many of her difficulties and was determined that the brain injury should not slow her down. She refused to pace herself. It was difficult to make tangible progress, but over a long period of time, Cathy began to speak more openly about her accident, remember more about her past and acknowledge some of her difficulties.

Denial

Denying that anything has changed allows the person to keep their old identity, which feels much safer, and may protect them from immediate distress and threat. However, the person may still feel anxious about not being able to live up to their old sense of self. They may be defensive and unwilling to discuss their brain injury. They will inevitably come across evidence of their brain injury difficulties, and find this hard to cope with.

Developing a new and more realistic sense of self is more difficult than denying the difficulties – but it allows a person to emerge on the other side in a more accepting and calmer state, with less need to fight against the injury.

How does this affect recovery and rehabilitation?

People become severely distressed if they do not have a stable sense of self or if they make negative 'then and now' comparisons. The distress may be expressed as depression; anxiety; anger; dependence on medication, drugs or alcohol; and suicidal thoughts.

Just as reduced self-awareness is a barrier to rehabilitation, it is difficult to engage in therapy or make efforts to improve if the person's identity does not include their stroke or brain injury.

Memory problems and other cognitive difficulties can affect the process of rebuilding identity. Building a new sense of self depends on remembering what has changed since the stroke or brain injury. Difficulties with self-awareness and flexible thinking can add to this.

I worked with a young man, Richard, who had no concept of the progress he had made since his severe brain injury. His mental health and adjustment to the injury were affected by this.

Richard believed that his life before the accident was perfect. He could not remember his serious injuries or how disabled he had been at first. He could not remember or 'see' the huge progress he had made over several years. He could only compare then (before the accident) and now.

If Richard could have appreciated the progress he had made, his sense of self might have evolved over time and become more positive. This situation was frustrating for everyone involved – Richard was constantly angry and dissatisfied, and the people around him felt stuck and helpless.

Situations like this are almost impossible to change. The best I could do was to sit and absorb the anger and frustration, to be alongside Richard as he raged against the injury – and perhaps to help his family to do the same sometimes.

Summary

Cognitive and emotional brain injury changes can trigger an identity crisis for the injured person. People usually feel they have changed for the worse. In addition, the changes don't fit with their stable, longstanding sense of self. The person has to try to make sense of this distressing difference between then and now.

The person no longer has a sense of who they are. The loss of this sense of self can create anxiety, confusion, sadness and anger.

One way out of the situation is denial, but this can cause many other problems in the long run. A positive way forward is for the person to become aware of and acknowledge their difficulties (if they have not already done so), to try to make sense of them and to include their difficulties and their brain injury in an updated identity that fits with their 'new normal'. This can be a long and painful process, which may require professional and family support.

Jody's altered sense of self

Jody did not have a strong sense of self in the early months. She knew she was a different person, and this was a 'terrible loss' in itself (Chapter 6). She had lost the sense of continuity within her own life.

Jody noticed many times that she was a different person now. The experience of that change would have been difficult to describe in words. There were hints of what Jody felt – for example, she could not respond to her colleagues as she used to. She could not answer questions quickly or fluently, or deal with more than one at a time (Chapter 12).

Jody lost her sense of self partly because she lost memories of her earlier life and her knowledge of the world. Our past and what we know define important parts of who we are. We build our identity and sense of self over the years by constantly updating it to include new memories, knowledge and experience. Losing some of this can fragment the sense of self, removing parts of the whole picture.

We use our memories, knowledge and experience to inform and guide how we behave. Jody turned to this vast library of information for answers, but 'there was little there – most of it had been eradicated, buried, moved or changed'. Feeling empty and without content was a part of Jody's changed sense of self (Chapter 2).

Jody felt alone in her relationship with herself. Her familiar sense of self was not there – 'I was not with me' (Chapter 2). Jody was more inclined to stay away from people when she felt like this, which was another change in who she was.

Jody tried to be the person she was before, to behave as she thought she would have done. She did things 'as if I was the same as before – but all the time I was an imposter' (Chapter 6). She could not be genuine when she was trying to be her old self. At the same time, being her new self was also difficult.

She had more sense of self when she was with other people. It gave her 'a sense of my identity… them and me… but on my own in those early months, I was anchorless' (Chapter 6). At other times, and particularly after the second stroke, being with people had the opposite effect.

Disconnection from the world

Jody 'knew two things – one, that I was different – and that I did not live in the world I had been in before – I was surrounded by it but somehow not in it' (Chapter 3). Jody had changed and the world seemed to have changed, too. Like a new and unfamiliar place, Jody could not find her way around it any more.

She observed that, 'It is hard to be without identity' and 'that was what I was doing, reinventing myself' (Chapter 5). She feared losing the poems she had learned, or losing 'the person I am now – go[ing] into a sort of no person land' (Chapter 10).

Jody describes herself as a ghost throughout her writing – a ghost of herself, or a ghost walking among people rather than really being with them. People could not see her as she really was, and she felt invisible. Jody described putting on a disguise so that no one could see the ghost that she was.

Old notebooks which she found but could not remember were like the notebooks of ghosts from the past. Jody's memory problems disconnected her from her past self, which had also become invisible (Chapter 21).

Connecting with Jody's old sense of self

The new version of a person's identity will never be completely different, and this continuity is essential for creating an acceptable and joined up 'story of me'. Jody was delighted when she discovered she still had some old skills – the tapestry, dancing the waltz and learning poetry: 'they connected me to old knowledge, the me that seemed to have gone' (Chapter 5).

At times, Jody had a strong sense of connection with her old self. Just before the second haemorrhage, she was doing better at work and regaining confidence in her abilities. 'At last I really felt BACK' (Chapter 13). The second stroke removed this connection with her old self for the second time – another reason why it was so painful.

Rebuilding a sense of self

Jody found she liked different things, particularly after her second stroke. This may have come partly from the brain injury changes. Jody's decision to declutter and to decorate the whole of her house with the same neutral colour was partly about the sensory overload she felt at home.

But it also came from a stronger sense of Jody knowing herself. Quite a long time after the second stroke, Jody commented: 'I could not live comfortably in my old environment. Where my old life was on display – with colour schemes that did not belong to the ME I am now' (Chapter 15).

Jody portrayed her changed sense of self most clearly with another powerful visual image. 'I am a brightly coloured rainbow jumper but someone unravelled it. And then if I knitted it again it would look the same on the surface but of course would be different, subtly different' (Chapter 4).

Jody's self-awareness and sense of self

A person with a brain injury can only begin to develop a new sense of self if they are aware of their difficulties. The changes must be recognised before they can be included in the new identity. Jody's mild self-awareness problems would have made this process slower and more difficult for her – coming up against problems that Jody did not expect or anticipate would have made her less sure of who she was.

Things that can help

Responding to the change

People with a brain injury often feel they have changed as a person. This may come from the way they feel inside, or from comparisons they make between themselves as they are now and how they were before.

It can be very difficult to admit to feeling changed, to being a different person. It brings out anxiety and alarm in everyone. We all want people to stay as they were.

Despite the difficulty involved, doing everything possible to acknowledge that the person feels different is important. Telling them that this is not unusual after a stroke or brain injury can be very reassuring.

Then and now comparisons

While 'then and now' comparisons are often painful and difficult, they are an important part of the adjustment process. They can be used as an opportunity to recognise and acknowledge how the person has changed, to build a new self-concept.

The comparisons need to be realistic. If the person says that they 'can't do anything now', they are probably feeling overwhelmed. Hearing themselves make sweeping generalisations will make them feel worse. If possible, help them to think more realistically about their difficulties and what they can do.

Some people tend to dwell on these comparisons for a long time, going round and round, unable to move on. The person with the injury may need help to be released from this cycle. Ideas and suggestions about improving the person's life should be mixed with understanding and sympathy for the pain, anger and difficulty they are experiencing.

Group support

Brain injury education and support groups can help people to make sense of their limitations and rebuild identity. Being part of a group allows people to share their experiences and to realise that difficulties with identity are normal. Watching other people go through the same process, especially people who are further ahead, can be very valuable. Groups can help to foster self-awareness, a more integrated sense of self and a stronger connection with other people.

Anxiety and what may help

Any change in our identity or sense of self is alarming and confusing. It often creates severe anxiety for the person who feels changed.

A person who feels changed may also feel disconnected and detached from themselves, the people around them and the outside world. They may feel remote, or see things as if through a veil or mist. This can be the brain's way of dealing with severe anxiety.

The most helpful way to respond to feeling changed, and to feeling anxious about it, is to focus on what is happening at this moment. Anxiety is usually about the future – the natural worries and concerns about being able to cope with life after a stroke or brain injury. Feeling threatened or diminished by the changes often adds to these.

Focusing on what is happening now, on breathing, and letting go of worrying thoughts and feelings about the future can help. Learning to relax can also reduce the anxiety.

Chapter 37: Acceptance

Moving towards acceptance after a stroke or brain injury

Moving towards acceptance is an important part of any recovery and rehabilitation journey. Accepting a brain injury is about owning the difficulties, as well as being able to recognise that they exist. Acceptance cannot develop without self-awareness of the difficulties, but acceptance is more than awareness alone.

Acceptance of a stroke or brain injury is about being willing to include it as part of a new identity, e.g. being able to say, 'My memory has been terrible since my brain injury'. It can also involve trying to make progress and improve things – being able to say, 'My memory has been terrible since my brain injury, and so I use reminders on my mobile phone to help me with this'.

We can't find a way around difficulties unless we acknowledge that we have them – to ourselves as well as to others. And so we cannot begin to make the best of a situation until we have begun to move towards an acceptance of it.

Acceptance as a journey

Moving towards acceptance after a severe brain injury is a long and often difficult journey. Acceptance isn't really an endpoint or a goal, but an ongoing, often unending process, with its own ups and downs, twists and turns.

Moving towards acceptance is an essential part of coming to terms with the injury. Developing greater acceptance can lead to changes in attitude and behaviour, including engagement in rehabilitation. The person who has become more accepting of their injury may be more willing to attend therapy sessions or practice things at home.

Jody's journey of acceptance

Jody's trek across the rope bridge and into the woods was a journey towards acceptance. She brought acceptance to her everyday experience of difficulty from the beginning. Her ability to stay with and to accept her experience came from her mindfulness practice, and had been part of her life before the stroke.

Despite this, it was often hard for her to bring acceptance to her difficulties. The natural inclination is to push unpleasant experiences away, rather than to accept them as simply another kind of experience. It is normal for people to dislike and to reject their limitations, to want things to be different, and especially to want things to be as they were before.

Part of Jody's acceptance was her realisation that she 'could not go back. The past was closed' (Chapter 5). As she became more certain of this, Jody began to let go of what was lost, and brought acceptance to her new reality. However she was now, she would 'live in this world as I am' (Chapter 4).

Jody found benefits in acceptance. She found that falling memories were more likely to return if she let them go. She appreciated small pleasures that came from not striving to be as she was before. She knew that wanting things to be different, hoping things would go away or pushing them away, would only deepen her distress and suffering, and keep them going for longer.

Even when things were difficult Jody found that she could accept things more easily when she stayed close to her present moment awareness. She knew that just as everything in life passes, unpleasant experiences would pass too.

She found acceptance in the present moment. If we can stay with things as they are, rather than struggle or turn away from them, being with them may help us to accept them. If we start to worry about them instead, we are trying to stop them happening, to avoid and protect ourselves from them. When Jody stayed focused on the present moment at difficult times, she was less likely to worry about what would happen next – and this was generally very helpful.

In difficult and overwhelming situations, Jody learned not to blame herself for her difficulties. This was another part of her acceptance.

Jody's acceptance after her second stroke

Jody wrote almost nothing about acceptance for a while after the second stroke. The positive and accepting part of Jody seemed to have been lost for a while in the woods.

Her accepting attitude seemed to return with her acceptance of the Wolves of Love and Hate. She wrote about the kindness of not striving to change things and 'just allowing ourselves to be as we are'. She was able to let memories go more easily, by thanking them for visiting and wishing them well (Chapter 16).

She began to see her difficulties as gateways rather than limitations, as openings into a new world where there was also beauty, and where she could let go of what had been lost.

Acceptance in mindfulness and rehabilitation

Mindful acceptance is about being with whatever is there. In rehabilitation, the same willingness to accept the difficulties as they are is seen as a gateway to adjustment and adaptation, towards making the best of what there is. Stroke and brain injury rehabilitation is rarely about trying to make a complete recovery, and it is important to be realistic about this.

Most of us do not have Jody's longstanding ability to turn towards difficulty. Nevertheless, learning to adopt a more accepting attitude can help in the aftermath of a stroke or brain injury. If it is at all possible, families can encourage acceptance in their relative by being more accepting themselves.

Problems with acceptance

Denial and avoidance

We all have a tendency towards non-acceptance. We deny things – 'it can't be true' – or push them away – 'I can't stand this'. We may cope by saying 'I just don't think about it' – we can be like the ostrich with its head in the sand.

Not thinking about the injury can make things seem better at first. But avoidance makes things worse in the long run. Not dealing with something doesn't make it go away. Blocking out sadness, anger and pain can eventually lead to depression and anxiety, rather than making us feel better.

A person who does not accept their brain injury difficulties can be puzzled when things go wrong – why is everything so difficult? What will go wrong next? Anxiety can start to creep in and trigger avoidance – perhaps using drugs, alcohol or self-harm to make the feelings go away. Sadly, alcohol and substance abuse problems are not unusual among people with a traumatic brain injury.

People may feel pessimistic about their recovery and be frightened to try things. They fear that they won't make progress. Concerns and uncertainty about the future, the 'what if' questions, can stop us in our tracks. What if I don't get better? What if I try and I can't do it?

People may think about this in black and white terms, with nothing grey in between. They may either expect complete failure or a full recovery. Unrealistic expectations can be difficult for everyone to work around.

Acknowledging problems can be very difficult

Some people believe that they don't need any help and that they do not need to change or adapt to their injury. They may believe that accepting help or using aids will interfere with their natural recovery.

A person who cannot accept their brain injury may make light of their difficulties, or may try to hide their problems. They may ignore advice, or be angry and aggressive when people talk about their problems, or when the difficulties become obvious to others.

Wishful thinking also works against acceptance – when people believe that what they wish for has actually happened. They may be focused on the past, on their life before the injury, and unable to think positively about the future.

What makes acceptance easier?

The people who accept their brain injury most easily could be described as more flexible. Younger people, people with more self-awareness and people who are motivated to improve their situation are more accepting. These people are usually more organised and better equipped to make changes and adjustments. People who were resourceful and good at coping with change before their injury also tend to be more accepting.

Changes caused by the brain injury can make acceptance more difficult. Problems with memory, reasoning and flexible thinking can reduce understanding and acceptance. To some extent, people with more severe injuries tend to be less accepting.

Difficulties with acceptance tend to go hand in hand with reduced self-awareness, or with strong emotional reactions to the brain injury, such as avoidance, anger, denial and blame. This is often part of a generally difficult situation – perhaps involving relationship difficulties, social isolation or being unable to work.

Being willing to adapt and make changes

Being willing to make the best of things involves acceptance. And as we have seen, moving towards acceptance is often a huge challenge. People may not be ready to admit that they would benefit from help or using aids, e.g. special kitchen gadgets, or a planning and memory board. Aids can be an unwanted reminder of their injury or disability, and they might rather struggle in the kitchen or forget things than use the aids.

Not wanting to be seen as disabled can also be an obstacle on the journey towards acceptance. People may avoid using aids in public for fear of drawing attention, being labelled or ridiculed. They may expect others to make negative remarks about their disability. A person who cannot accept their own difficulties cannot imagine other people accepting them either. Anxiety and unshakable beliefs around these issues can mean that opportunities are lost and life is less fulfilling.

On a more positive note, the benefits of beginning to use aids can trigger a positive cycle that allows the person to do more, and to accept more help.

Fighting with the injury

Some people can get locked in a battle with the effects of their stroke or brain injury. They feel it would be weak to accept the changes, and they refuse to give in to the brain injury or let it beat them. They may rage against the unfairness of the situation or the person who caused it.

This kind of battle can be difficult to change, especially if the person is inflexible or has reasoning difficulties. The fight with the brain injury may be a very important part of their lives. For example, they may fight endlessly to be allowed to manage their own finances, unable to accept that they do not have the mental capacity to do so.

Acceptance is not a straight path

The path towards acceptance tends to twist and turn. Psychological denial can come and go. Denial can be helpful sometimes, and even encourage acceptance in the long run. It may protect a person from despair and despondency, for a while at least. Unexpected changes, such as a new friend or a new activity, can allow more acceptance to develop.

Ian was sure that he had recovered fully after a severe stroke. He fought against having more help at home. The more upset and frustrated he felt, the more he denied his difficulties. Despite this, Ian sometimes talked quite openly about his problems.

This only ever happened towards the end of our afternoon sessions. Being listened to made Ian feel calm and safe enough to 'admit' to them. Unfortunately, his chaotic family life did not make him feel safe or listened to, and it was many years before he could acknowledge or begin to accept his severe difficulties when he was with his family.

Fault and blame – another obstacle to acceptance

We often try to work out why things happen, to find reasons for them, and perhaps to find something to blame. This may also hinder acceptance.

Brain injuries are sometimes caused by someone else, who can then be blamed for the injury. Strokes can be caused by medical mistakes or negligence. The injured person may have been assaulted, or hurt in a road accident that was not their fault. In this situation, people often feel that they did not deserve what happened to them, which is perfectly true. No one 'deserves' a stroke or brain injury.

Many injuries are the result of bad luck, of random events beyond anyone's control. Occasionally, however, an injury is caused by an accidental drug overdose, a suicide attempt or risky behaviour such as driving when drunk. The person may feel that they only have themselves to blame. Moving towards acceptance of this very sad situation is particularly difficult, and encouraging the person to talking about how they feel would be even more important.

Acceptance is more difficult when an injury was avoidable or appears to be another person's fault.

Moving forward towards acceptance

Acceptance of a brain injury involves a gradual understanding and allowing of what has happened. It leads to a willingness to 'be with' it and to find ways around it, whatever the cause was. Accepting that the injury cannot be changed is an important step, even if that brings more distress in the short term.

Acceptance does not mean feeling happy or okay about the situation. You can accept that something difficult has happened, and feel sad or angry about it at the same time. It does not mean that what happened was right. It involves saying that it happened and that these are the consequences.

It is important to emphasise that acceptance is never an end point, something that is achieved, put aside and forgotten about. It is an ongoing process of remembering the injury, experiencing its effects, incorporating it into the 'same but different' sense of self, and feeling more comfortable with not trying to control it or push it away.

Acceptance is most clearly expressed through a willingness to try to improve the situation. If a person does not accept their difficulties, trying to persuade someone to change what they do can be an uphill struggle.

People can move towards greater acceptance through the process of trying something new and succeeding with it. Persuading the person to work towards achievable goals can be an important step forwards. It can be the start of a process in which they feel more confident and more comfortable about acknowledging their difficulties.

Finding meaning in loss and injury

Moving towards acceptance can be easier if the person or their family can find some meaning in the changes and losses caused by the brain injury.

Surviving a stroke or brain injury can feel like having a second chance. Despite the difficulties involved, people may see it as an opportunity to rethink their values and direction in life. They may be able to do things that they always wanted to, but they did not have time for before.

There can be meaning in the new pace of life after a brain injury. Life in the 'slow lane' can be valuable in a different way and more fulfilling. There may be more time to spend with wider family and friends, and fewer stressful expectations of success and achievement.

Some people make sense of their injury through their religious or spiritual beliefs. They may believe that the injury happened for a reason. They may want to use their pain and difficulty in the service of their religion, or to help others.

How the injured person makes sense of their loss will depend on the kind of person they were before. It will also depend on the difficulties they have now. If at all possible, it can be helpful to see beyond the brain injury and to think about other aspects of their life.

The person may have valuable strengths and abilities to offer. Using these to do things that they enjoy or to help others can foster a sense of achievement and stronger links with the community, increase self-esteem and help in the journey towards acceptance.

Things that can help

What's the worst that can happen?

A small amount of progress is good enough. Try to chase away perfectionism and unrealistic expectations.

If you feel reluctant to try something out, it can be helpful to write down the advantages and costs of doing it (or not doing it). You may find that the risks are not high and that you enjoy it more than you expect.

It may be helpful to remember that you won't know unless you try. You are much more likely to make a small amount of progress than to fail.

You could try something on the understanding that you can stop if you want to after an certain time (or number of attempts).

The future is uncertain

If you feel anxious about the future, it might help to focus on what is happening now. Anxious feelings are based on our thoughts and imagination. Thoughts and images are just thoughts and images – they are in the mind, and the mind is not the same as reality.

The future is uncertain for everyone, and worrying about it, or assuming that it will be a certain way, does not change things or make them any better. There is often more health and contentment to be found in the present moment.

If you are interested in developing the ability to focus more on the present moment, you might choose to try a mindfulness practice. Jody has recorded some of the mindfulness practices she used since her brain haemorrhage – a link to these is in the Practices section on page 305. There are also mindfulness apps, and other recorded practices available on the internet and in mindfulness books.

continued >

One day at a time

Fear and anxiety about the future often involves a long-term view. Focusing on today, tomorrow or next week, where there is more certainty, can be reassuring and calming. Taking one day at a time removes that frightening distant future perspective.

Remembering that Rome wasn't built in a day and that recovery and progress take time might help to ward off impatience or the desire to give up. The slow and steady approach in the Hare and the Tortoise story is a good way to think about this.

Understanding and acceptance

A better understanding of their brain injury can encourage a person's acceptance. Books and films about brain injury, or attending education groups with similar people, can also encourage acceptance. Absorbing some information and being part of the group where others are more accepting may lead to small positive changes.

Planned failure

Very occasionally, it is acceptable for a person to attempt something that no one else believes they can do. Someone who does not accept a widely held opinion that they would not be able to drive safely might nevertheless have driving lessons and perhaps a driving test. This may sound harsh or unfair, but sometimes the person may only believe independent feedback.

A failed test may encourage other options, such as taxis or public transport, and allow the issue to be put to rest. The person is likely to need a lot of emotional support to cope with the failure, but in the right circumstances, a stuck situation can be transformed into a learning experience.

Feedback and realistic hope

Feedback about failure illustrates a person's difficulties. The right kind of feedback can foster acceptance of them. Better still, positive feedback about the gains the person has made is invaluable for acceptance.

It is important to be positive and hopeful, but at the same time, to recognise that setbacks are inevitable. They are easier to cope with if you know they might happen and are prepared for them. This involves balancing hope and optimism with realistic judgements.

A wider perspective

If it seems appropriate, it can be useful to shift the focus slightly away from the brain injury. The brain injury must be there, of course, but as part of a larger picture – that includes other parts of the person and their life.

This can remind the person of opportunities that have been ignored until now and might be tried. It can be easier to move towards acceptance when the brain injury does not occupy the whole landscape, and is surrounded by other more positive aspects of life.

continued >

> **Mindful acceptance**
>
> Being more mindful in daily life and through meditation practice can help to manage stress.
>
> Taking a few moments to sit and breathe, as Jody so often did in moments of difficulty, can recharge our batteries enough to move on.
>
> Deliberately adopting an attitude of acceptance, acknowledging that this is how it is (whether I like it or not), rather than trying to push away sad or anxious thoughts and feelings, can also be very helpful in the long run.
>
> Many people with a brain injury struggle to adopt some of the mental perspectives involved in mindfulness practice, e.g. noticing thoughts or noticing links between thoughts and feelings. As mental flexibility and self-awareness are often affected by a stroke or brain injury, these complex cognitive manoeuvres are likely to be too difficult for people with a severe injury.
>
> Nevertheless, people with a stroke or brain injury can become more aware of their surroundings, of their breath, of sensations in their body, and can benefit from this as much as anyone else. Learning to practice mindfulness is known to help people with a traumatic brain injury who are also depressed or anxious.
>
> As Jody has shown so clearly, a long-term mindfulness practice can help a person to accept and deal with the frustration, loss and anxiety that a brain injury causes.

An overview of the journey

The journey from a brain injury towards acceptance and adjustment is often long and tough for everyone involved. It involves a number of different stages, although these can overlap and blur into each other. People may go backwards and forwards between stages, or, in the saddest of situations, they may get stuck and not move towards an acceptance of their situation at all. Working with a psychological therapist can sometimes help when people are stuck, or when they can't get started.

In order to begin the journey, the person with a brain injury must have some awareness of their difficulties, particularly their cognitive, emotional and behavioural changes. This may include a sense of being a different person. Becoming more aware of these changes often leads to sadness and despair, and wanting the situation to go back to 'normal'. It is important that the person experiences and understands the link between their sadness and the things they have lost.

Expressing sadness, anger, bewilderment and despair about the changes can be very difficult and exhausting. However, grief is an important part of coming to terms with the brain injury. If the emotions are 'bottled up' or the person does not know why they feel so unhappy, the feelings will probably come out in more harmful ways. This could be anything from destructive rage, to drinking heavily, to self-harm and feeling suicidal.

The journey also involves making sense of what has happened. It may be a bit like a jigsaw puzzle, slowly creating a bigger picture of how the person is, what they can and cannot do now, and what the future may look like for them. Some of this may be explored in rehabilitation therapy – for example, physiotherapy and occupational therapy. These are designed to improve the situation, but they also bring the injured person into contact with their limitations.

Time is important here – so often described as a great healer. Spending time being focused on the difficulties, with people (including rehabilitation therapists) who are kind and supportive and who can help to improve function, can lead to a sense of the 'new normal' that Jody wrote about. This process of emotional adjustment could almost be described as making sense of it and gradually becoming more used to it.

Making sense of a brain injury and the problems it has caused can be extremely challenging. The person may have lost some of the abilities they need to make sense of things, and the intensity of the emotions that can take over when things do not make sense can be frightening and unpleasant.

Making sense is partly about understanding what has happened. Another part is about finding meaning in the difficult changes, and in the way life may be in the future. This might involve thinking about what is important to the person now – their values and what they want their life to be about. It can involve thinking more broadly, about important things in life that are not the brain injury – for example, an interest in sport, volunteering, family life or religion.

Adjusting to a brain injury involves building a 'same-but-different' sense of self or identity. All of these stages are important on a journey that moves towards acceptance. Together they can lead to a willingness to be with things as they are, rather than only wanting them to be as they were, a willingness to make changes and progress, and to live a different kind of life.

Chapter 38: Families

Family care after a stroke or brain injury
Jody did not need as much family support as many people do. She was able to carry on living alone, and after a few months, she needed relatively little outside help.

Families and caregiving
Families often play an essential role in care and rehabilitation after a stroke or brain injury. Most people with a brain injury return home to live with their family, who may then become the person's caregivers.

Finding out what the injury means for the family
When the person comes home from hospital, there is often huge relief about their survival and recovery so far. The family is often called upon to rearrange their lives quickly, and to support their relative. However, there are likely to be more challenges ahead. Less visible brain injury changes may emerge, and the family may not know how to cope with the new situation.

Families find it more difficult to cope with personality, behavioural and emotional changes than with even severe physical disabilities, or memory and other cognitive problems. These difficulties strike at the heart of family relationships.

Relationship changes
The difficulties that affect family relationships can vary widely. Mild changes in attitude, self-centredness and lack of concern can be as disturbing as more obvious or severe changes, such as aggression or inappropriate behaviour. In some families, the injured relative may seem to be less likeable and more difficult to be around. Difficult behaviour may need to be understood and even 'managed' by the family.

When personality changes affect core family relationships, there are huge emotional losses. For a partner, the loss of mutual love, attention and intimacy can be devastating. Spouses who once shared their concerns and supported each other through thick and thin can become quite separate, emotionally.

Children who support a parent with a brain injury go through a distressing role reversal as they become a caregiver, and often have emotional problems. They can no longer depend on the parent to look after them, and they can feel abandoned and isolated.

Taking on a new role

Family members may have to take on new roles and responsibilities. They may have to take over cooking, gardening or managing household finances from the injured person. The person may need help with personal care and daily tasks including dressing, transport, communication and remembering to do things.

If the person with a stroke or brain injury has had to give up work, a family member may also have to leave their job, and there may be a considerable financial loss. Some families make significant lifestyle changes, which is stressful in itself.

It can be difficult to balance the needs of the injured person and the needs of the family. We have become more aware of the needs of families in recent years, and brain injury rehabilitation often includes family support.

The family can do a lot to support their injured relative and to improve their situation. However, caring for a person with a brain injury can be challenging, tiring and stressful. Families need help and support in order to take care of their own physical and mental health.

How family members can help their injured relative

Families can support their injured relative best by understanding them as much as possible. This may sound obvious or even simple, but it can take enormous skill and judgement, at a time when the family may already feel exhausted or at a low ebb. Understanding as much as possible about what makes the person tick, and acting as their advocate, can make an enormous difference.

Understanding difficult behaviour

People with a brain injury often express feelings of confusion, sadness, loss, anger and frustration in words and actions that are difficult for others to cope with. The 'bad behaviour' brakes may be off, and their difficult feelings may just tumble out. The injured person may lash out or blame their family for their injury and difficulties. If this happens regularly, it can wear away at the family's patience and ability to cope.

The challenge is to try to understand where the behaviour is coming from rather than taking it personally, or reacting to it at face value. Families sometimes fall back on their old rules of life. They may, quite understandably, feel like blaming the injured person, rather than trying to understand what lies behind the difficult behaviour.

The person may need help with controlling their emotions or impulsive behaviour, perhaps by making it clear that saying or doing some things are not acceptable, or developing strategies designed to increase the person's self-control. For example, a 'stop and think' or 'stop and take a deep breath' routine can be helpful.

If a caregiver can see that emotions are building up or that the person's behaviour is changing in a particular way, they may be able to use a special signal, agreed in advance, that means 'stop and think' or 'stop and breathe'. This may prevent situations escalating out of control.

Many stroke and brain injury changes can easily be misunderstood. Having no motivation, or no concern for others, or little self-awareness can all stem directly from the brain injury. The person might appear to be 'lazy', 'selfish' or 'manipulative' when, in reality, these changes are beyond their control.

Asking the person how they feel when they are behaving differently can be a good starting point. They may not be able to explain their behaviour, but they may be able to say how they feel. Being willing to listen and to understand may help both parties.

The person may be in pain, or feeling emotional about how they have changed and the situation they are in now. They may be feeling sad or anxious, bewildered and confused, and unable to put these feelings into words. Helping them begin to make sense of what has happened to them can be an important step forward.

Finding meaning and finding positives in change

Families may be able to find positives in the 'new normal', and to make the most of happier or more relaxed time together. A sense of humour and being able to laugh at things can also make a difference. Being positive can be difficult, but it can be infectious too. A deliberate decision to behave in a more positive way may help if you are beginning to feel dragged down by the situation.

Eventually, even families who have suffered great loss may find new meaning in the stroke or brain injury. Difficult experiences can bring families together.

Relatives and friends may see how important they are to each other, and spend more time together.

Surviving a medical emergency or serious accident can change the world view of both the survivor and their loved ones. Making a fresh start may be important for the whole family.

Elizabeth

A young woman with a brain injury and her father were recently interviewed on the TV. Elizabeth was 22 when she had a stroke, two years before the interview. She talked about what people need most from their families – understanding; patience, love and support; being positive, friendly and nice.

Having encouragement and a push at the right time was also important – Elizabeth's motivation could go up and down. She had joined various groups with the Stroke Association and Start, and found art therapy particularly helpful.

Elizabeth's dad said that it had been a very emotional time for the family. He recommended reaching out for any available help and support, from health services and voluntary groups.

Family grief and loss

When a brain injury changes a person's character and behaviour, families and close friends can feel the loss as though it were a bereavement.

Grief may not surface for many months or even years, until the family is sure that there will never be a complete recovery. This can be a very difficult point, where the family lets go of their fading hope for a return to the way things were. As caring is often a full-time, stressful job, the grief may also have to wait until the caregiver has the time and emotional strength to cope with the emotions triggered by this realisation.

Grief involves recognising the change and loss and allowing the sadness and distress to be experienced. It is an important part of coming to terms with life after a relative's brain injury.

The 'burden' of caregiving

We know that caring for a relative with a stroke or brain injury tends to become more difficult over time. At the same time, the caregiver plays a crucial role – an injured relative will be more content and have a better quality of life if their family is coping well.

This is a huge responsibility, and one that many families cannot carry on their own. Family caregivers need support and guidance in order to care well, especially as caring becomes more difficult over time.

Complex difficulties and relationship changes may mean that the family's mental health and coping skills are worn down. There may be a vicious circle, where stress and frustration for both the family and the injured relative rub off on each other, and they spiral down together. Many family caregivers are depressed or anxious or both, and are often very tired and stressed.

Strong families cope well

Families who lived happily together before the brain injury are often more resilient. Families who can say difficult things as well as positive things do better than families who don't communicate well. Families that work together to find ways around difficulties, have a positive attitude towards their injured relative and can even see benefits in change are happier and more united in the long run.

Families with unresolved or difficult past relationships, and families who are not well organised, often need more help when a family member has a stroke or brain injury.

What families need

Help and support from people outside the family can help to reduce the stress. This can range from a friend who comes in for a chat or who keeps an eye on things while the caregiver goes out, to professional help or involvement in groups of families who share their experience and wisdom. Being understood and supported by others can reduce the impact of changes such as difficult behaviour and poor self-awareness.

Family caregivers also benefit from information and education about stroke and brain injury, especially about how their relative has been affected.

Services and how they work

After leaving hospital, some patients and their families have access to community brain injury or stroke rehabilitation services. These provide longer-term support for people living at home. Services for traumatic brain injury and stroke are organised in different ways across the UK, and the amount of support available varies widely.

Stroke rehabilitation in hospital and at home tends to focus mainly on physical and practical problems – through physiotherapy, speech and language therapy and occupational therapy. Other services, designed for people with traumatic brain injury, strokes and other acquired brain injuries, are more likely to address cognitive and emotional changes as well. These are also more likely to involve the family in the rehabilitation and to provide support for families.

Understanding brain injury

Knowing more about their relative's brain injury and its consequences can improve the situation for the family. Therapists and other professionals often include families when they give feedback about a clinical assessment. This could be a physiotherapy, speech and language, occupational therapy or neuropsychology assessment. Understanding what the problems are, where they come from and which difficulties seem to be improving can help the family to understand their situation and how best to help.

Brain injury and stroke education groups for families can also be very helpful. These are often run through specialist brain injury services. Voluntary sector groups such as Headway and the Stroke Association also run family groups and encourage families to share information and experiences.

Sharing experiences and advice with people in the same boat helps families to feel less alone, and to realise that their reactions are normal. It may help them to feel less guilty – and to blame themselves less – for being upset, stressed or angry with their relative.

There are many books and leaflets about the effects of a stroke or brain injury, and how best to cope with the difficulties. Reading these or joining a group as early as possible can help to prevent crises and overwhelming problems. There is a short Further Reading list on page 308.

A brain injury is as difficult for the family as it is for the injured person. This is now so well recognised that specialised therapies have been developed to help families adjust and adapt as well as possible.

Cycles of stress

The problems faced by families are often more complex than they seem. We usually see the brain injury as 'the problem', and so fixing things for the injured person can appear to be the best way forward. Sometimes, the problem may be more about how everyone, including the injured person, reacts to the situation.

Some families need to be closely involved and to protect their relative with a stroke or brain injury from risk. However, this can make change and movement towards greater independence more difficult in later stages. The involvement may need to become more flexible.

Chris, who was in his early thirties, had lived with his parents since he had a traumatic brain injury (TBI) in a car accident at the age of 15. He had severe memory problems and fatigue, and was quite volatile emotionally. He also had very severe epilepsy that did not respond to medication. He was more likely to have a seizure when he was tired.

His mother was very protective of Chris, and was particularly anxious about him doing too much and triggering more seizures. The seizures knocked Chris out of action for several days afterwards and aggravated his memory problems.

Chris worked part time in a supported recycling workshop, alongside his girlfriend, Lucy, who also had a TBI. Chris and Lucy wanted to live together but Chris's mother was against it. She did not think that Lucy could cope with the seizures or look after him properly afterwards.

His mother thought that living away from home would be too much for Chris and that the fatigue would make the seizures worse. There were many arguments about this.

The team involved in Chris's care negotiated with Chris and his parents, and eventually Chris rented a flat nearby. Chris and Lucy gradually spent more time there. Eventually, they lived together full time, except for one night a week, which Chris spent at his parents' house. Chris was more settled and had fewer seizures. His mother, who lived half a mile away, was able to look after him when he had one.

For other families, the situation can improve when they become more involved.

Steve was a middle-aged man with young children who had suffered a severe stroke almost a year before. He was not enjoying his therapy days at the rehabilitation centre and did not want to continue. He said they were a waste of time and just made him feel stupid. His wife, Jill, wanted him to carry on, but did not want them to 'cause trouble' by discussing his complaints with the therapists.

Steve's reluctance led to many arguments and eventually he refused to go to the centre at all. He called the centre with various excuses. Within a short time, he became less mobile and less motivated. He did less around the house and was impatient with the children. This deterioration was distressing for the whole family, and caused further tension between Steve and Jill.

After a few weeks, one of the therapists came to see Steve and Jill to ask about his attendance. It turned out that Steve's withdrawal was about the group of elderly men who attended on the same days. He felt patronised and misunderstood when he was treated in the same way as them. He would have preferred to be with people of his own age.

Steve also had unrealistic expectations of the therapy. He did not fully understand, and could not remember, what the therapy was intended to do.

Steve and Jill went into the centre for a meeting with some of the staff. The therapists explained Steve's difficulties and the basis of his therapy again, and gave Steve a written summary of this information. They said that Steve could attend on different days of the week, when there were a few other younger people coming in, and Steve agreed to start again. Jill began to pick him up at the end of the day so that one of the staff could fill her in about Steve's day.

Open communication between the person with the stroke, their family and professionals is often crucial. A conversation with one of the therapists when the problems first began might have helped Steve's wife and the rehab team to understand the situation better, and to provide Steve with the kind of approach that would have kept him engaged.

In some stroke and brain injury services, couples or whole families can be seen together to talk through issues like this or relationship difficulties. Children with a parent who has a brain injury can go to activity and support groups that may help them to better understand what is happening at home.

The power of group support

I have worked with family groups in the health service and in Headway, and have seen how helpful it is for families to share their experiences. One group, called Working with Family Stress, was an eight week programme based on mindfulness and acceptance. Working with the families showed how difficult it is for caregivers to recognise and express their own feelings of sadness and grief. These feelings were often bottled up.

It was hard for the caregivers to look after themselves, and to sometimes put themselves first. Guilt, and anxiety about risk are often part of this. Relatives can feel trapped in a literally self-less role, that can lead to burnout, anger and resentment. This is an understandable trap to fall into. Addressing it can help the family to recover a meaningful life together.

This approach does not try to stop feelings of loss and sadness. These are natural and important. It does not try to 'fix' the stroke or brain injury, either. Instead, it aims to help people live better and be happier in the situation as it is. Moving towards an acceptance of the situation and learning to live with the long-lasting effects of the injury can help the family cope better, care better and be more resilient.

The take home message is that we can't control difficult events in life, or the way they make us feel. But we can decide how to respond to those feelings

– whether we let them control us, or whether we move forward with those feelings on board.

The family groups were based partly on the idea that what is good for the family is good for the injured relative. Families often feel that they can't improve their difficult situation or escape from it. Developing more acceptance of their own feelings about the injury, while learning to take care of themselves and reduce their own stress, can help families to come to terms with the situation.

Summary

Looking after a relative with a brain injury is often difficult and demanding, both emotionally and physically. It tends to become more stressful over time. Changes in the person's behaviour and emotions cause the most stress.

The whole family benefits when caregivers understand the brain injury changes, particularly when they involve difficult behaviour or emotions. Information and education are very important. It is much easier to support a relative if their behaviour, emotions and injury as a whole make sense and are understood.

Caregivers need to look after themselves, too. In practice, this can be difficult. Family members may feel guilty because they seem to be putting their own needs before the needs of their relative. However, it is essential for families to look after themselves in order to look after their relative.

> ### Things that can help
> #### Supporting a relative with a stroke or brain injury
> Families can do a lot to assist in their relative's recovery. Providing emotional support, security and encouragement can make all the difference.
>
> Make the most of what the person can do and avoid things that emphasise their difficulties. Try to include and involve them as much as possible, allowing them to feel useful and an important part of the family – not only someone who needs to be looked after.
>
> How you feel and behave will affect your injured relative – in a positive way or negatively. If there is a problem, try to see whether you are a part of it, and whether changing something might help.
>
> Be as positive as possible and enjoy happier moments as they happen. Even if you don't feel like it, putting on a brave face and a smile can be helpful.
>
> Reading about stroke and brain injury can be helpful, especially if you don't have access to rehabilitation.
>
> Don't expect to be a perfect caregiver, or to do everything you did before. Try not to blame yourself if you get things wrong. It is a steep learning curve.
>
> continued >

Difficult behaviour and emotions

Difficult behaviour may be the expression of difficult emotions. Families can help by trying to understand what this behaviour means and what the distress is about.

Try to talk to the person with the injury about how they are feeling and what might be wrong. Listen carefully, without interrupting. They may be in pain, or exhausted or upset about their stroke and difficulties.

Try to understand the person's behaviour. They may not be able to control what they say or do. At the same time, be clear that some behaviours are not acceptable. Develop a 'stop and think' or 'stop and breathe' plan.

Doing even simple things may be difficult for the person with a brain injury. They may take time and a lot of energy, or be painful or frustrating. You may need a lot of patience.

Looking after yourself

You need to look after yourself to be able to look after someone else.

You may benefit from some professional support or counselling if you are feeling low in mood or anxious. You may need help to grieve or to let go of the past.

Allow yourself to grieve, to cry and feel sad. This is a healthy and important part of coming to terms with the loss. It can be good to think about the past and to remember happier times – look at photos, share the memories with your relative if possible. People sometimes feel that they should avoid reminders of the past, but it will help you all to remember what you are grieving for.

It can be very difficult to meet your own needs as well as the needs of your injured relative. You may feel under constant pressure to be caring in some way, or this pressure may come from yourself. Try not to feel guilty about time off. It's important.

Ask for help or respite when you need it. Don't wait for a crisis.

Spend as much time with friends and other family as you can. Invite people to the house so that the whole family is involved.

It will be harder to do things for yourself if the person you care for wants you to be there all the time. They might feel anxious about losing you in some way. Reassure them and build up your time away slowly, so that they feel more confident. Plan your outings ahead of time, so the person expects it and has everything they need.

Do things that you enjoy – a massage or a swim, meeting friends or going for a walk in the park. Time for you should be about recharging your batteries rather than getting things done. Have a weekly routine for your own time, and stick to it.

Talking with other families and people who understand can be very valuable. You might join a group for stroke or brain injury families, or another type of family care group. This may help you to feel less alone and isolated.

Expect to feel sad and perhaps angry about the situation. Talk about this; don't bottle it up. Working through these feelings may help you to cope better in the long run, to find new ways of doing things and solving problems.

Take one day at a time, and try not to worry too much about the future.

The Unseen

Here, now, at what seems like the end of all things –
I feel the stir and movement of my breath –
As though great wings of Angels are near...
Calling me to Let Go... to allow myself to trust...
To rest in the cracks between light and dark
Where day and night merge.
The place where peace and fear meet...
Where all things – like the breath...
Turn... and Turn again.
(Jody Mardula)

Jody's practices

Audio recordings of these mindfulness practices can be downloaded from: https://www.pavpub.com/mindfulness-and-stroke-resources

Hands practice

I felt the sense of my hands resting on the sheets.
I could feel the softness of the sheets beneath the hands.
Breathing into the hands.
And deliberately imagined the sense of hands.
The remembered sense of their hands resting on mine.
Lying there, on my raft bed, breathing into my hands.
Connected, I was not alone.

Grounded breathing practice

Notice the contact of my body with the sheets
Feel the weight of my body against the bed – supported
Bring my attention to the movement of the in breath and the out breath
Feeling the sensation of the breath in the nostrils and the mouth
The rise and fall of the belly with the breath
Letting go of any tension
Dropping into just lying there breathing
And noticing any thoughts
Seeing if I could just allow them to pass
Not getting caught up in worries and thoughts
But just resting there, breathing in and out
For a few moments.

The cup practice

I take my spacious cup or bowl and sit on a chair, or bed, or anywhere I am supported.
And I bring my attention to my body sitting here.
Feel the contact of the body on the seat/bed/chair
And feel the contact of my hands holding the cup.
And I bring attention to my breath
Following and noticing the in breath and out breath.
Allowing this to be a space to rest and just let be –
As if held and cradled by the cup.
Allowing the ups and downs and difficulties that may be here.

Walking practice

Noticed the contact of my feet with the ground on each step
I am counting them, step one, step two,
And I breathe into each step,
Breathing in, breathing out
Bringing the attention into just this moment,
Letting go of all the thoughts.
And just being in this moment of walking.

Grounding and settling practice

GROUND yourself.
Just become aware of the body, either feet on floor… maybe feet walking, or body sitting on a chair or a bench.
Noticing whatever the contact points are – and feeling them – the weight of the body. In contact with the ground or the seat.
And becoming aware of your breathing, just noticing and following as you breathe in and out. Nothing else to do. Just aware of being here. Of breathing. And then perhaps remembering whatever is going on, to think of yourself kindly. Ah, this is tough – I am tired – I don't know what to do… just acknowledging whatever is here for you, and be kind as you might be to a child, or a loved other. And notice and allow the movement of your breath, in and out of the body.

A breathing space

STOP – whatever you are doing, wherever you are – either just standing still, or going to sit somewhere, anywhere – on a bench, in a café or in your meditation space.

SIT – and bringing attention to asking WHAT IS HAPPENING NOW?
Just NOTICING – what is there in your body – sensations – in your mind – thoughts coming and going.

BREATHING – following my in breath and out breath – this breath, this breath, this breath.
LETTING GO of whatever is here and just simply following the breath – and GROUNDING – that sense of the body solid, here, sitting on my seat.

This might be a brief 3–5 minute practice – or even just a few moments, or longer, if you like, depending on time and circumstances.

Settling with difficulty practice

Taking your seat,
Adopting an upright posture,
Letting the eyes close and hands rest comfortably on the lap.
Becoming aware of the contact and weight of the body on the cushion or chair.
Becoming aware of the posture of the whole body, the weight going down and the height going up
The head reaching up toward the sky.

Watching and feeling the in breath and the out breath.
Just sitting and breathing.
This breath all the way in… this breath all the way out
And if the mind wanders off as minds do,
Just coming back to the body sitting here
And the breath moving in, moving out.

And as we sit we may notice thoughts and feelings come up
So not trying to do anything with them,
Not hanging on or pushing away.
With an attitude of gentle kindness towards yourself
Just sitting and breathing.

And if pain, or worrying thoughts, or difficulty arise in the body
Then as best you can do not push them away or try to avoid them
But sit and breathe allowing even this to be here.
Sitting.

A soft owl practice

Holding something soft like a soft toy in the hand, and squeezing in and then letting go, squeezing in and then letting go.
Directing the attention to the sensation of squeezing and then the sensation of loosening your hold on the little soft owl… and then beginning to include the breath.
Noticing the in breath as you feel the pressure of your hand squeezing the toy and then the out breath as you release… rather than trying to force your tired brain to think 'in breath and out breath', let your hand do it for you.

Squeezing and breathing in, releasing and breathing out.
Squeezing and breathing in, releasing and breathing out.

No need to think about the hand squeezing and releasing, or the breath, breathing in and breathing out – just let it be a natural thing to squeeze and breathe.

Further reading and useful organisations

Living with stroke and brain injury
Bolte Taylor J (2009) *My Stroke of Insight*. London: Hodder.

McDonald S, Little A & Robinson G (2019) *Rebuilding Life After Brain Injury: Survivor stories*. London: Psychology Press.

Morris R, Falck M, Miles T, Wilcox J & Fisher-Hicks S (2017) *Rebuilding Your Life after Stroke*. London: Jessica Kingsley Publishers.

Powell T (2004) *Head Injury: A practical guide*. Abingdon: Speechmark Publishing.

About the brain
Goldberg E (2009) *The New Executive Brain: Frontal Lobes in a Complex World*. Oxford: Oxford University Press.

Passingham R (2016) *Cognitive Neuroscience: A Very Short Introduction*. Oxford: Oxford University Press.

Sacks O (1986) *The Man Who Mistook His Wife for a Hat*. London: Picador.

Siegel D (2007) *The Mindful Brain: Reflection and Attunement in the Cultivation of Well-Being*. London: W.W. Norton.

Mindfulness
Kabat-Zinn J (2005) *Wherever You Go, There You Are: Mindfulness Meditation in Everyday Life*. Westport: Hyperion.

Williams M & Penman D (2011) *Mindfulness: A Practical Guide to Finding Peace in a Frantic World*. London: Piatkus. Contains a CD of guided meditations.

Dementia
McCurry S (2008) *When a Family Member Has Dementia: Steps to Becoming a Resilient Caregiver*. Santa Barbara: Greenwood World Publishing.

Voluntary sector organisations
SameYou: For brain injury recovery – https://www.sameyou.org. The actress Emilia Clarke's (who also suffered a subarachnoid haemorrhage) organisation which aims to raise awareness and increase access to rehabilitation for adults with brain injury, including younger people.

Stroke Association – www.stroke.org.uk

Headway – www.headway.org.uk

Alzheimer's Society – www.alzheimers.org.uk

Other references

Aniskiewicz A (2007) *Psychotherapy for Neuropsychological Challenges*. Lanham: Jason Aronson.

Bowen C, Yeates G & Palmer S (2010) *A Relational Approach to Rehabilitation: Thinking about Relationships after brain injury*. London: Karnac Books.

Coetzer R (2006) *Traumatic Brain Injury Rehabilitation: A Psychotherapeutic approach to loss and grief*. Hauppage: Nova Science Publishers.

Coetzer R (2010) *Anxiety and Mood Disorders Following Traumatic Brain Injury*. London: Karnac Books.

Gurd J, Kischka U & Marshall J (2012) *The Handbook of Clinical Neuropsychology*. Oxford: Oxford University Press.

Hayes S, Follette V & Lineham M (2004) *Mindfulness and Acceptance: Expanding the cognitive-behavioral tradition*. New York: The Guilford Press.

Leclerq M & Zimmerman P (2002) *Applied Neuropsychology of Attention: Theory, diagnosis and rehabilitation*. London: Psychology Press.

Klonoff P (2010) *Psychotherapy after Brain Injury: Principles and techniques*. New York: The Guilford Press.

Lezak M, Howieson D & Loring D (2004) *Neuropsychological Assessment* (4th edition). Oxford: Oxford University Press.

Ponsford J, Sloan S & Snow P (2017) *Traumatic Brain Injury: Rehabilitation for everyday adaptive living* (2nd edition). London: Psychology Press.

Sherer M & Sanders A (2014) *Handbook on the Neuropsychology of Traumatic Brain Injury*. Berlin: Springer.

Wilson B, Gracey F, Evans J & Bateman A (2009) *Neuropsychological Rehabilitation: Theory, models therapy and outcome*. Cambridge: Cambridge University Press.